The
Gut-Brain
Connection

Overcoming Ulcerative Colitis
Through
Mindfulness And Nutrition

Grace N.I

LZR Publications and Press

176 New Umuahia Road, Aba

Abia State

Chizaramnnachi2000@gmail.com

Grace N.I

First Edition

Disclaimer:

This book is not intended to be a substitute for medical advice or treatment, any person with condition requiring medical attention should consult with a qualified medical practitioner or suitable therapist. The information provided in this book is stated to be truthful and consistent, in that any liability, in terms of inattention or otherwise, by any usage or abuse of any policies, processes, or directions contained within is the solitary and utter responsibility of the recipient reader. Under no circumstances will any legal responsibility or blame be held against the publisher for any reparation, damages, or monetary loss due to the information herein, either directly or indirectly.

TABLE OF CONTENTS

Dedication ... 8

Acknowledgement ... 9

Preface ... 10

PART ONE

Introduction to Ulcerative Colitis ... 12

CHAPTER ONE

What Is Ulcerative Colitis? ... 14

- ❖ Types of ulcerative colitis ... 14
- ❖ Causes of ulcerative colitis ... 15
- ❖ Symptoms of ulcerative colitis ... 20

CHAPTER TWO

Foods to avoid and foods to eat ... 22

- ❖ Bread and starches ... 22
- ❖ Meat and protein ... 24
- ❖ Vegetables ... 25
- ❖ Fruits ... 27

PART TWO: Recipes ... 29

CHAPTER THREE: Breakfast ... 31

- ❖ Soup of butternut squash ... 31
- ❖ Sweet potato ginger pancakes ... 33
- ❖ Apple and banana pancakes ... 35
- ❖ Cake lemon bars ... 37

❖	Orange and honey duck	39
❖	Sweet potato, egg and avocado breakfast	41
❖	Ginger bread waffles	43
❖	Smoked salmon frittata	45
❖	Egg bake	47
❖	Chocolate zucchini muffins	49
❖	Breakfast berry crisp	51
❖	Golden overnight oat with orange flavor	53
❖	Blueberry pancakes with oatmeal	55
❖	Green peanut butter-banana smoothie	57
❖	Mediterranean eggplant shakshuka	59
❖	Frittatas with spinach and red peppers	61
❖	Avocado-egg salad toast	63

CHAPTER FOUR: Lunch — 66

❖	Chicken lettuce wraps	66
❖	Beef skewers	68
❖	Roasted pumpkin curry	70
❖	Shrimp maple skewers	72
❖	Pan-seared scallops	73
❖	Shrimp tomato salad	74
❖	Tomato salmon bowl	75
❖	Ground chicken with tomatoes	76
❖	Beef and veggie burgers	77
❖	Eggs and avocado endive wraps	78
❖	Greek cucumber salad	79
❖	Beef and spinach burgers	80
❖	European beet soup	81
❖	Pasta with asparagus	82
❖	Turkey burgers	83
❖	Pasta with zucchini and tomatoes	84
❖	Beef and mozzarella burgers	85

❖ Tuna stuffed avocado	86
❖ Shrimp lettuce wraps	87
❖ Lemony scallops	88

CHAPTER FIVE: Dinner — 91

❖ Stuffed zucchini boats	91
❖ Chicken cutlets	93
❖ Halibut curry	94
❖ Rosemary chicken	95
❖ Lemony salmon	96
❖ Herb salmon	97
❖ Cantaloupe gnocchi	98
❖ Veggie risotto	99
❖ Lemon pepper turkey	100
❖ Chicken piccata	101
❖ Whole roasted trout	102
❖ Turkey and kale sauté	103
❖ Winter apple poke bowl	104
❖ Prawn and tomato spaghetti	106
❖ Chicken cacciatore	107
❖ Peach stew	109
❖ Shrimp and salmon tomato stew	110
❖ Zero-fibre chicken dish	112
❖ Brazilian fish stew	114
❖ Turkey with rosemary	115
❖ Grilled salmon steaks	116
❖ Fiesta chicken tacos	117
❖ Shrimp scampi pizza	118

CHAPTER SIX: Desserts — 120

❖ Vegan pecan tart with chocolate crust	120
❖ Vegan granola cups	122

- ❖ Dairy-free and gluten-free carrot cake   124
- ❖ Dairy-free banana chocolate ice cream   126
- ❖ Gluten-free and dairy-free blueberry cupcakes   127
- ❖ Vegan and gluten-free chocolate hazelnut spread   129
- ❖ Vegan and gluten-free tofu chocolate cakes   130
- ❖ Vegan and gluten-free pink lemonade cupcakes   132
- ❖ Autumnal vegan carrots with walnuts   134
- ❖ Java bananas   135
- ❖ Sweet dessert bliss   136
- ❖ Gluten-free and dairy-free apple crumb   137
- ❖ Dairy-free custard   138
- ❖ Fried honey bananas   139
- ❖ Avocado sorbet   140
- ❖ Banana cupcakes   141
- ❖ Flourless chocolate cake   142
- ❖ Eggless honey cake   143
- ❖ Christmas in a cup   145
- ❖ Brownie bites   147
- ❖ Blueberry galette   148
- ❖ Royal crown pie   150
- ❖ Mocha ricotta crème   152
- ❖ Orange muffins   153

CHAPTER SEVEN: Snacks   157

- ❖ Cookie cup tarts   157
- ❖ Fruit and ginger popsicles   158
- ❖ Yogurt bites   159
- ❖ Baked mushroom snacks   160
- ❖ Chili chickpeas   161

❖ Peanut butter snack   162

❖ Pita snacks   163

❖ Cheesy potato frittata   164

❖ Haystack yummy   166

❖ Crispy rice snacks   167

❖ Gluten-free trail mix   168

❖ Coconut balls   169

❖ Buffalo chicken dip   170

❖ Chocolate chia balls   171

❖ Sweet potato hummus   172

❖ Zucchini chips   173

❖ Caramel energy bites   174

❖ Coconut tofu tenders   175

❖ Falafel   176

❖ Swede (rutabaga) chips   178

❖ Spicy pineapple salsa   179

❖ Angel hair pasta with lemon and parmesan   181

❖ Nice cream sundae   182

❖ Garden frittata   183

PART THREE: MEAL PLAN   186

CONCLUSION   190

DEDICATION

This book is dedicated to all those who live with ulcerative colitis. You are the inspiration for this book. Your courage, determination and resilience in the face of this challenging disease have been an inspiration to us all. We hope that this book will provide you with the information and support you need to better understand and manage your condition.

We also dedicate this book to your families and loved ones, who provide unwavering support and understanding.

May this book be a source of hope and encouragement for you on your journey towards healing and wellness.

ACKNOWLEDGEMENTS

We would like to express our deepest gratitude to all the individuals who have contributed to the creation of this book. First and foremost, we would like to thank the patients who have shared their personal stories and experiences with us. Their courage and willingness to share their journey has been invaluable in providing insight and inspiration for others.

We are also grateful to the healthcare professionals who have provided their expertise and guidance throughout the research and writing process. Their dedication and commitment to improving the lives of those affected by ulcerative colitis has been an inspiration.

We would also like to extend our thanks to our colleagues, friends and family for their support and encouragement. This book would not have been possible without their unwavering belief in our work.

We are grateful to the publisher for their support and guidance throughout the publication process.

And finally, we would like to express our heartfelt appreciation to our readers, who have taken the time to read this book. We hope that it will serve as a valuable resource for anyone impacted by ulcerative colitis

PREFACE

Ulcerative colitis is a chronic and debilitating condition that affects the large intestine and rectum. It is a form of inflammatory bowel disease (IBD) that causes inflammation, ulceration and bleeding in the colon and rectum. Despite significant advances in medical treatment and surgical options, the disease remains a significant challenge for patients and their families. The physical, emotional, and social impact of ulcerative colitis can be devastating, and the search for effective therapies is ongoing.

This book is a guide for anyone affected by ulcerative colitis, including patients, family members, and healthcare professionals. It covers a wide range of recipes and recommended foods for UC patients, as well as practical advice for managing symptoms and improving quality of life. The book is divided into several chapters, each one focusing on a specific approach and diet for managing ulcerative colitis. The first chapter provides an overview of the disease, including its causes, symptoms, and diagnosis. The following chapters delve deeper into the various foods that help to keep the disease in check.

The book includes a vast section on nutrition and diet, and the recipes to prepare such foods which can be an important factor in managing ulcerative colitis.

Finally, the book concludes with a section on the emotional and social impact of ulcerative colitis.

We hope that this book will serve as a valuable resource for anyone impacted by ulcerative colitis, and we are honored to have the opportunity to share this information with you. Whether you are a patient, a family member, or a healthcare professional, we believe that this book will provide you with the information and support you need to better understand and manage the disease.

-**Zaram N.N**

Co-author

PART ONE

INTRODUCTION TO ULCERATIVE COLITIS

Ulcerative colitis is a relatively common condition worldwide, with an estimated 1.6 million people affected in the United States alone. The exact prevalence of ulcerative colitis varies by region, but it is estimated to affect approximately 0.1% to 0.2% of the global population. The incidence of ulcerative colitis is higher in developed countries than in developing countries, with the highest rates reported in North America and Europe.

In general, the incidence of ulcerative colitis is higher in people of white European descent, but the condition can affect people of any race or ethnicity. It tends to be more common in people who are of Northern European descent, and it's less common in people of African or Asian descent. It affects men and women equally.

Ulcerative colitis is a chronic condition that affects the large intestine and rectum. It is a form of inflammatory bowel disease (IBD) that causes ulcers and inflammation in the lining of the colon and rectum. Symptoms of ulcerative colitis can include abdominal pain, diarrhea, and rectal bleeding. The condition can have a significant impact on a person's quality of life and can lead to serious complications if left untreated.

This book provides a comprehensive guide to understanding ulcerative colitis, including its causes, symptoms, diagnosis, and treatment options. It also covers practical tips for managing the condition and coping with the emotional and psychological impact it can have. Whether you are a patient, a family member, or a healthcare professional, this book is an essential resource for anyone seeking to better understand and manage ulcerative colitis

CHAPTER ONE

What Is Ulcerative Colitis?

Ulcerative colitis is a chronic inflammatory bowel disease (IBD) that causes inflammation and sores in the innermost lining of the colon (large intestine) and rectum. It causes inflammation, ulceration and bleeding in the affected area, and can lead to a variety of symptoms, such as abdominal pain, diarrhea, and rectal bleeding.

Ulcerative colitis forms a range from mild to severe. If left unchecked, it can lead to life-threatening complications and it puts the patient at increased risk of developing colon cancer. There are no cure for ulcerative colitis, but it can be managed with medications, surgery, and life style changes.

TYPES OF ULCERATIVE COLITIS

Ulcerative colitis is often classified according to its location by health care providers.

They include:

Proctosigmoiditis; This type of ulcerative colitis involves the inflammation of the rectum and the lower end of the colon. The patient have symptoms such as abdominal cramps, diarrhea, and inability or extreme difficulty in bowel movement despite the urge to do so.

Ulcerative proctitis; In a case of ulcerative proctitis, the inflammation is only in the area closest to the anus, which is the Rectum. The only well-known symptom of Ulcerative proctitis may be rectal bleeding.

Pancolitis; Patients with Pancolitis often have severe bloody diarrhea, fatigue, abdominal pain and cramps, and a significant weight loss. Pancolitis usually affect the entire colon.

Left-sided colitis; In Left-sided colitis, inflammation extends from the rectum up, through the descending portions of the large intestine.

Symptoms of left-sided colitis include abdominal cramps and pain on the left side, bloody diarrhea, and urgency to defecate.

CAUSES OF ULCERATIVE COLITIS

Although the exact cause of ulcerative colitis is yet unknown, diet and stress were suspected in the past. However, we know today that these factors may aggravate but not cause ulcerative colitis.

With recent discoveries coming to light, we know a number of factors that can cause ulcerative colitis:

An excessive immune function:

It is believed that Ulcerative colitis is caused by an abnormal immune response in the gastrointestinal tract (GIT). The exact mechanism by which this occurs is not fully understood, but it is thought to involve an overactive immune system that causes inflammation in the colon and rectum.

Normally, the immune system helps to protect the body from harmful invaders, such as bacteria and viruses. In people with ulcerative colitis, the immune system mistakenly attacks the cells in the lining of the colon and rectum, leading to inflammation and ulceration.

It is thought that this abnormal immune response may be triggered by a combination of genetic, environmental, and lifestyle factors. Some research suggests that a combination of genetic predisposition and an environmental trigger, such as a viral or bacterial infection, may lead to the development of ulcerative colitis. Other studies have suggested that certain lifestyle factors, such as diet, stress, and smoking, may also contribute to the development of the condition.

In summary, the excessive immune function is thought to cause ulcerative colitis by mistakenly attacking the cells in the lining of the colon and rectum, leading to inflammation and ulceration. The exact cause of this abnormal immune response is not fully understood, but it is likely to involve a combination of genetic, environmental, and lifestyle factors.

Genetics:

Genetics is believed to play a role in the development of ulcerative colitis. Studies have shown that the risk of developing the condition is higher in people who have a family history of the disease. It's estimated that about 10-

15% of people with ulcerative colitis have a first-degree relative (parent, sibling, child) with the disease.

Research has identified several genetic variations that are associated with an increased risk of developing ulcerative colitis. Some of these variations are in genes that are involved in the immune system and may play a role in the abnormal immune response that leads to inflammation in the colon and rectum. Other genetic variations are associated with the regulation of the gut micro biome.

It is important to note that genetics is only one of the factors that contribute to the development of ulcerative colitis. The condition is also thought to be caused by a combination of environmental and lifestyle factors. For example, research has suggested that certain environmental triggers, such as viral or bacterial infections, may increase the risk of developing ulcerative colitis in people who are genetically predisposed to the condition.

In summary, while genetics is believed to play a role in the development of ulcerative colitis, it is not the only factor. Environmental and lifestyle factors also contribute to the development of the condition, and more research is needed to fully understand the complex interplay between genetics and the environment in the development of ulcerative colitis.

Environmental factors:

Environmental factors are believed to play a role in the development of ulcerative colitis. The exact environmental triggers that may contribute to the development of the condition are not fully understood, but several factors have been proposed.

One theory is that a viral or bacterial infection may trigger an abnormal immune response that leads to inflammation in the colon and rectum. Studies have suggested that certain viruses, such as the cytomegalovirus, may be associated with an increased risk of developing ulcerative colitis.

Another theory is that changes in the gut microbiome, or the community of microorganisms that live in the gut, may contribute to the development of ulcerative colitis. Research has suggested that imbalances in the gut microbiome, such as an overgrowth of certain bacteria or a lack of beneficial bacteria, may play a role in the abnormal immune response that leads to inflammation in the colon and rectum.

Another environmental factor is diet. Studies have shown that certain dietary habits and food items may be associated with an increased risk of developing ulcerative colitis, such as a high intake of processed foods, saturated fats, and red meat.

Other factors that have been proposed include stress and smoking. Stress has been linked to a flare-up of symptoms in people who already have the condition, while smoking has been linked to an increased risk of developing the disease.

It is worth noting that while environmental factors may play a role in the development of ulcerative colitis, it is not fully understood how these factors interact with genetics, it's also likely that different environmental factors may play a role in different people. More research is needed to fully understand the complex interplay between genetics and the environment in the development of ulcerative colitis

Micro biomes of the gut:

The gut microbiome refers to the community of microorganisms that live in the gut. Research has suggested that imbalances in the gut microbiome, also known as dysbiosis, may play a role in the development of ulcerative colitis.

Studies have shown that the gut microbiome of people with ulcerative colitis is different from the microbiome of healthy individuals. Specifically, people with ulcerative colitis tend to have a lower diversity of gut microorganisms, and a higher proportion of certain types of bacteria, such as Proteobacteria and Firmicutes, compared to healthy individuals.

It is thought that these imbalances in the gut microbiome may contribute to the abnormal immune response that leads to inflammation in the colon and rectum. For example, certain bacteria may produce inflammatory compounds that can damage the lining of the gut, or they may affect the immune system in a way that causes it to attack the cells in the colon and rectum.

Research has also suggested that the gut microbiome may play a role in the response to treatment in ulcerative colitis. Studies have shown that after treatment, the gut microbiome of people with ulcerative colitis tends to become more similar to the microbiome of healthy individuals, and this may be associated with an improvement in symptoms.

It's worth noting that the research on the gut microbiome and ulcerative colitis is still ongoing and more research is needed to fully understand the complex interactions between the gut microbiome and the development of ulcerative colitis. However, it is becoming clear that the gut microbiome plays an important role in the disease and targeting the gut microbiome may be a potential therapeutic strategy for ulcerative colitis.

SYMPTOMS OF ULCERATIVE COLITIS

- Rectal bleeding
- Diarrhea
- Urgency to defecate
- Rectal pain
- Abdominal pain and cramping
- Inability or extreme difficulty to defecate despite urgency
- Fatigue
- Fever
- Cases in children may lead to stunted growth

CHAPTER TWO

Foods To Avoid And Foods To Eat

A patient with ulcerative colitis should aim to have a balanced diet that is high in nutrient-dense foods, while avoiding foods that may exacerbate their symptoms. The specific recommendations for bread and carbohydrates may vary depending on the individual and the severity of their condition. However, some general guidelines include:

BREAD AND STARCHES:

Allowed foods;

- **Whole grains:** Whole-grain breads, cereals, and pasta can provide important nutrients and may be easier to digest than refined grains.
  Examples include whole wheat bread, oats, quinoa, brown rice, and barley.

- **Gluten-free options:** Some people with ulcerative colitis may find that gluten-free options such as rice, corn, and quinoa breads, pasta, and cereals are easier to digest.

- **Low-Fiber options:** High-fiber foods can be difficult to digest and may exacerbate symptoms in some people with ulcerative colitis. Low-fiber options include white bread, pasta, and rice, which may be easier to tolerate during a flare-up.

Foods to avoid;

Some people with ulcerative colitis may find that certain foods, such as spicy foods, processed foods, and high-fat foods, can exacerbate their symptoms.

Other foods to avoid include;

- **High-Fiber options:** High-fiber foods can be difficult to digest and may exacerbate symptoms in some people with ulcerative colitis. High-fiber options include whole grain breads, cereals, and pasta, as well as fruits and vegetables with tough skins or seeds.

- **Gluten-containing options:** Some people with ulcerative colitis may find that gluten-containing options such as wheat bread, pasta, and cereals can be difficult to digest and exacerbate symptoms.

- **Certain fermented foods:** Some fermented foods such as sourdough bread, pickles, sauerkraut may contain high levels of histamine which can cause flare-ups in some people.

- **Certain nuts and seeds:** Some people with ulcerative colitis may find that nuts and seeds, such as almonds, cashews, and sunflower seeds, can be difficult to digest and may exacerbate symptoms. It's worth noting that each individual may have different tolerance level, and it's important to work with a dietitian or a healthcare provider to develop a personalized dietary plan that works best for the individual. They can help to determine which foods are best to avoid during a flare-up and which foods to eat. Additionally, it's important to remember that some foods that may be problematic for one person with UC may be well-tolerated by another, so it's essential to pay attention to how your body reacts to different foods.

MEAT AND PROTEIN:

The specific recommendations for meats and proteins may vary depending on the individual and the severity of their condition. However, some general guidelines include:

Allowed foods:

- **Lean meats:** Lean cuts of meats such as chicken, turkey, fish, and lean cuts of beef and pork can be a good source of protein and may be easier to digest than high-fat meats.

- **Plant-based protein sources:** Plant-based protein sources such as beans, lentils, tofu, and tempeh are also good options and may be easier to digest than some animal-based protein sources.

- **Low-fat dairy:** Low-fat dairy products such as milk, yogurt, and cheese can provide important nutrients such as calcium and protein, but it's important to choose low-fat options to avoid exacerbating symptoms.

- **Eggs:** Eggs can be a good source of protein and easy to digest for some people.

Foods to avoid:

- **High-fat meats:** High-fat meats such as fatty cuts of beef, pork, and lamb, as well as processed meats (such as bacon, sausages, and deli meats) may be difficult to digest and may exacerbate symptoms.

- **Certain seafood:** some seafood such as shellfish and oily fish (salmon, tuna, and sardines) may cause flare-ups in some people with ulcerative colitis.

- **Certain processed foods:** Some processed foods such as frozen dinners and fast food can be high in fat, sodium, and other additives that can be difficult to digest and may exacerbate symptoms

VEGETABLES:

Allowed foods:

- **Soft cooked vegetables:** Soft cooked vegetables such as spinach, zucchini, eggplant, bell peppers, and tomatoes may be easier to digest than raw vegetables.
- **Low-Fiber options:** High-fiber vegetables can be difficult to digest and may exacerbate symptoms in some people with ulcerative colitis. Low-fiber

options include mushrooms, white potatoes, and carrots.

- **Leafy greens:** Leafy greens such as lettuce, kale, and arugula are also good options and can provide important nutrients.

- **Squash and pumpkin:** These vegetables can be well tolerated by some patients with UC.

Foods to avoid:

- **High-Fiber options:** High-fiber vegetables can be difficult to digest and may exacerbate symptoms in some people with ulcerative colitis. High-fiber options include broccoli, cauliflower, Brussels sprouts, and kale.

- **Legumes:** Some legumes such as beans, lentils, and peas may be difficult to digest and may exacerbate symptoms.

- **Certain raw vegetables:** Some raw vegetables such as raw onions, raw garlic and raw peppers may cause flare-ups in some people with ulcerative colitis.

- **Certain cruciferous vegetables:** Some cruciferous vegetables such as cabbage, broccoli, cauliflower and kale may cause gas and bloating which can exacerbate symptoms in some people with ulcerative colitis.

FRUITS:

Allowed foods:

- Watermelon
- Peach
- Plum
- Apricot
- Papaya
- Honeydew
- Banana
- Nectarine
- Cantaloupe

Foods to avoid:

All dried fruits, fruits with pulp or seeds, berries, and generally high-fiber fruits.

PART TWO

<u>RECIPES</u>

The recipe provided is generally considered safe for people with ulcerative colitis, as long as they are able to tolerate the ingredients used. However, it's always best to consult with a physician or a registered dietitian to get personalized advice, as different people with ulcerative colitis may have different dietary needs. As you know, Ulcerative colitis is a type of inflammatory bowel disease (IBD) that causes inflammation and sores, or ulcers, in the lining of the rectum and colon. People with this condition often experience symptoms such as diarrhea, abdominal pain, and rectal bleeding, and may have difficulty tolerating certain foods.

In general, a diet for people with ulcerative colitis should be low in fat and high in fiber, to promote regular bowel movements and reduce inflammation. Some people may find it helpful to avoid foods that are high in sugar, gluten, or spicy ingredients.

Butternut squash is a good source of fiber, vitamins, and minerals, and is considered to be a gentle food that is easy to digest. However, some people with ulcerative colitis may have difficulty tolerating high-fiber foods, or may need to limit their intake of certain fruits and vegetables due to a condition called "pouchitis".

If you have ulcerative colitis or any other health condition, please consult with a healthcare professional before making any significant changes to your diet.

CHAPTER THREE

Breakfast

SOUP OF BUTTERNUT SQUASH

Here is a recipe for a simple butternut squash soup:

Ingredients:

- 1 large butternut squash, peeled and diced
- 1 onion, diced
- 2 cloves of garlic, minced
- 4 cups of vegetable broth
- 1 cup of heavy cream (optional)
- Salt and pepper, to taste
- Olive oil, for cooking
- Fresh thyme or sage, for garnish (optional)

Directions:

- In a large pot or Dutch oven, heat a drizzle of olive oil over medium heat. Add the diced onion and cook until softened, about 5 minutes.
- Add the minced garlic, cook for about another minute.
- Add the diced butternut squash, broth, salt, and pepper to the pot.

- Bring the mixture to a boil, then reduce the heat and let simmer for 20-25 minutes or until the squash is very tender.
- Use an immersion blender or transfer the soup to a blender and blend until smooth.
- If using, stir in the heavy cream.
- Taste and adjust seasoning as you desire.
- Ladle the soup into bowls and garnish with fresh thyme or sage, if desired.
- You can enjoy this soup as it is or you can add some toppings of your preference.
- Enjoy your meal!

SWEET POTATO GINGER PANCAKES

Here's a recipe for sweet potato ginger pancakes:

Ingredients:

- 1 cup of cooked and mashed sweet potato
- 1 egg
- 1/2 cup of milk
- 1/2 cup of flour
- 1 tsp of baking powder
- 1 tsp of ground ginger
- 1 tsp of cinnamon
- 1/4 tsp of salt
- 1 tbsp of brown sugar (optional)
- Butter or oil, for cooking

Directions:

- In a medium bowl, combine the cooked and mashed sweet potato, egg, and milk. Mix well.
- In another bowl, combine the flour, baking powder, ginger, cinnamon, salt, and brown sugar (if using). Mix well.
- Add all the dry ingredients to the wet ingredients and stir until the mixture is evenly combined.
- Heat a skillet or griddle over medium heat and add a small amount of butter or oil.
- Scoop or pour about 1/4 cup of batter per pancake onto the skillet or griddle.
- Cook for 2-3 minutes on each side or until golden brown and cooked through.

- Repeat the same procedure with the remaining batter.
- Serve the pancakes with your favorite syrup or toppings.

Sweet potatoes are a good source of vitamins, minerals, and antioxidants, and they also provide a natural sweetness to the pancakes. Ginger adds a nice spicy note and it's also known for its anti-inflammatory properties. This recipe is gluten-free, but you can use wheat flour as well.

As always, if you have any dietary restrictions or allergies, please consult with a healthcare professional before making any significant changes to your diet.

<u>APPLE AND BANANA PANCAKES</u>

Here is a simple recipe for apple and banana pancakes:

Ingredients:

- 1 cup all-purpose flour
- 2 teaspoons baking powder
- 1/2 teaspoon salt
- 1/2 teaspoon ground cinnamon
- 1 egg
- 1 cup milk
- 2 tablespoons melted butter
- 1 medium banana, mashed
- 1 medium apple, peeled and grated

Directions:

- In a large mixing bowl, combine the flour, baking powder, salt, and cinnamon.
- In a separate bowl, beat the egg and add the milk, melted butter, mashed banana, and grated apple. Mix well.
- Pour the mixture of the wet ingredients into the dry ingredients and stir until it is evenly combined.
- Heat a griddle or non-stick pan over medium-high heat.
- Using a ladle or measuring cup, pour the batter onto the pan or griddle.
- Cook until bubbles form on the surface and the edges start to look set, then flip and cook until golden brown.

- Serve with maple syrup and butter if desired.

CAKE LEMON BARS

Here is a recipe for lemon cake bars:

Ingredients:

Crust:

- 1 and 1/2 cups all-purpose flour
- 1/2 cup powdered sugar
- 1/2 cup unsalted butter, room temperature

Filling:

- 4 large eggs
- 1 and 1/2 cups granulated sugar
- 1/4 cup all-purpose flour
- 3/4 cup fresh lemon juice
- 2 tablespoons lemon zest
- 1/4 teaspoon salt

Directions:

- Preheat your oven to 350°F (175°C) and grease a 9x13 inch baking pan.
- In a medium mixing bowl, combine the flour and powdered sugar. Cut in the butter using a pastry cutter or your fingers until the mixture resembles coarse crumbs. Press the mixture into the bottom of the prepared pan.
- Bake the crust for 15-20 minutes or until lightly golden brown. Remove from oven and let it cool.

- In a large mixing bowl, beat the eggs, granulated sugar, flour, lemon juice, lemon zest, and salt together until well combined. Then pour the mixture over the crust that is already cooled.
- Bake the lemon bars for 25-30 minutes or until the filling is set. Remove from oven and let it cool to room temperature.
- Dust with powdered sugar before cutting and serving.
- Lemon bars are a delicious dessert that can be enjoyed with a cup of tea or coffee.

Keep in mind that, as mentioned before, people with Ulcerative Colitis may have to avoid certain foods that can aggravate their symptoms, and it's always best to consult with a healthcare professional or a registered dietitian who is familiar with your condition, as they can give you personalized advice on what foods to include or avoid in your diet.

<u>ORANGE AND HONEY DUCK</u>

Here is a recipe for Orange and Honey Duck:

Ingredients:

- 4 duck breasts
- Salt and pepper
- 1/4 cup honey
- 1/4 cup orange juice
- 2 tablespoon soy sauce
- 1 tablespoon rice vinegar
- 1 teaspoon grated ginger
- 1 clove garlic, minced
- 1/4 teaspoon red pepper flakes (optional)
- 1 orange, thinly sliced
- 1/4 cup fresh parsley, chopped (optional, for garnish)

Directions:

- Preheat oven to 375°F.
- With pepper and salt, season the duck breasts.
- In a small saucepan, combine the honey, orange juice, soy sauce, rice vinegar, ginger, garlic and red pepper flakes, if using. Heat over medium-high heat, stirring occasionally, until the sauce thickens, about 5 minutes.
- Over medium-high heat, heat a large skillet. Add the duck breasts, skin-side down, and cook for about 3-4 minutes per side, or until the skin is golden brown and crispy.

- Remove the skillet from heat and brush the duck breasts with the honey-orange sauce.
- Arrange the orange slices on top of the duck breasts and transfer the skillet to the preheated oven.
- Bake the duck for about 8-10 minutes, or until the internal temperature of the duck reaches 145°F.
- Remove the skillet from the oven and let the duck rest for a few minutes before slicing.
- Garnish with chopped parsley, if desired, and serve with the remaining sauce.

Note: Cooking times may vary depending on the size and thickness of your duck breasts. It's best to use a meat thermometer to ensure that the duck is cooked to your liking.

<u>SWEET POTATO, EGG AND AVOCADO BREAKFAST</u>

Here's a recipe for a Sweet Potato, Egg, and Avocado Breakfast:

Ingredients:

- 1 medium sweet potato, peeled and diced
- 1 tablespoon olive oil
- Salt and pepper
- 4 eggs
- 1 avocado, diced
- 1/4 cup diced red onion (optional)
- 1/4 cup chopped cilantro (optional)
- Lime wedges, for serving

Directions:

- Preheat your oven to 400°F.
- Toss the diced sweet potato in olive oil and season with salt and pepper.
- Arrange the sweet potato on a baking sheet and roast in the preheated oven for 20-25 minutes or until tender and golden brown.
- While the sweet potato is cooking, heat a skillet over medium heat then crack the eggs into the skillet and cook to the level of doneness you desire.
- Once the sweet potato is done, remove from the oven and assemble the dish. Divide the sweet potato, avocado, and eggs among plates.
- Garnish with diced red onion and chopped cilantro, if desired.

- Serve with lime wedges to squeeze over the top.

This dish is a great source of healthy fats and protein, it's gluten-free and can be enjoyed as a breakfast or brunch. You can add different vegetables or seasonings according to your preference.

<u>GINGER BREAD WAFFLES</u>

Here's a recipe for Gingerbread Waffles:

Ingredients:

- 2 cups all-purpose flour
- 2 teaspoons baking powder
- 1/2 teaspoon baking soda
- 2 teaspoons ground ginger
- 1 teaspoon ground cinnamon
- 1/4 teaspoon ground nutmeg
- 1/4 teaspoon ground cloves
- 1/2 teaspoon salt
- 2 eggs, separated
- 1 cup buttermilk
- 1/2 cup molasses
- 1/4 cup brown sugar
- 1/4 cup unsalted butter, melted
- 1 teaspoon vanilla extract

Directions:

- In a large mixing bowl, combine the flour, baking powder, baking soda, ginger, cinnamon, nutmeg, cloves, and salt.
- Beat the egg whites in a separate mixing bowl until stiff peaks form.
- In another mixing bowl, beat the egg yolks, buttermilk, molasses, brown sugar, melted butter, and vanilla extract until well combined.

- Pour the mixture of wet ingredients to the dry ingredients and mix until it is evenly combined.
- Fold in the beaten egg whites.
- Preheat your waffle iron according to the manufacturer's directions.
- Pour batter onto the waffle iron and cook until golden brown and crispy.
- Serve the waffles warm with butter and maple syrup.

These gingerbread waffles are perfect for the holiday season. They are full of warm spices and rich molasses flavor. You can also add some chopped nuts or dried fruits to the batter if desired, and also can be topped with whipped cream, fruits, or even caramel sauce.

SMOKED SALMON FRITTATA

Here's a recipe for a Smoked Salmon Frittata:

Ingredients:

- 8 eggs
- 1/4 cup heavy cream
- Salt and pepper
- 1 tablespoon olive oil
- 1/4 cup diced red onion
- 1/4 cup diced bell pepper
- 2 cloves garlic, minced
- 4 oz smoked salmon, diced
- 1/4 cup of grated Parmesan cheese
- 2 tablespoons chopped fresh dill (optional)

Directions:

- Preheat your oven to 350°F.
- In a mixing bowl, whisk together the eggs, cream, salt, and pepper.
- In a skillet over medium heat, add the olive oil, red onion, bell pepper and garlic. Cook for about 3-4 minutes or until softened.
- Add the diced smoked salmon to the skillet and stir to combine.
- Pour the egg mixture over the vegetables and salmon in the skillet, and cook over medium heat until the edges start to set, about 2-3 minutes.

- Sprinkle the grated Parmesan cheese over the frittata and transfer the skillet to the preheated oven.
- Bake the frittata for about 8-10 minutes or until the center is set and the top is golden brown.
- Remove the skillet from the oven and let the frittata cool for a few minutes before slicing.
- Garnish with chopped dill, if desired and serve warm.

This frittata is a great way to use up leftover smoked salmon and it's perfect for brunch or breakfast. It's also a great source of protein and healthy fats. You can also add some more veggies or cheese to make it more flavorful, or you can change smoked salmon to any kind of fish or seafood that you like.

<u>EGG BAKE</u>

Here's a recipe for an Egg Bake:

Ingredients:

- 8 eggs
- 1/2 cup milk
- Salt and pepper
- 1/4 cup diced ham or bacon
- 1/4 cup diced bell pepper
- 1/4 cup diced onion
- 1/2 cup shredded cheddar cheese
- 1/4 cup chopped fresh parsley (optional)

Directions:

- Preheat your oven to 350°F.
- In a mixing bowl, whisk together the eggs, milk, salt and pepper.
- In a skillet over medium heat, add the diced ham or bacon and cook until crispy.
- Remove the bacon or ham from the skillet and set aside.
- Add the diced bell pepper and onion to the skillet and sauté for about 3-4 minutes or until softened.
- Grease a 9x13 inch baking dish with cooking spray.
- Pour the egg mixture into the baking dish and top with the sautéed vegetables, cooked ham or bacon, shredded cheese.
- Bake in the preheated oven for 20-25 minutes or until the eggs are set and the top is golden brown.

- Remove the baking dish from the oven and let the egg bake cool for a few minutes before slicing.
- Garnish with chopped parsley, if desired and serve warm.

This egg bake is a great way to use up leftovers and it's perfect for brunch or breakfast. It's a great source of protein and you can add or change the ingredients according to your preference. You can add or switch out ingredients like diced mushrooms, spinach, or any kind of cheese.

CHOCOLATE ZUCCHINI MUFFINS

Here's a recipe for Chocolate Zucchini Muffins:

Ingredients:

- 1 1/2 cups all-purpose flour
- 1/2 cup unsweetened cocoa powder
- 1 teaspoon baking powder
- 1/2 teaspoon baking soda
- 1/4 teaspoon salt
- 1/2 cup granulated sugar
- 1/2 cup brown sugar
- 1/2 cup vegetable oil
- 2 eggs
- 1 teaspoon vanilla extract
- 1 cup grated zucchini
- 1/2 cup semisweet chocolate chips

Directions:

- Preheat your oven to 350°F. Grease a muffin tin or line with muffin cups.
- In a mixing bowl, combine the flour, cocoa powder, baking powder, baking soda, and salt.
- In another mixing bowl, beat the granulated sugar, brown sugar, oil, eggs, and vanilla extract until well combined.
- Stir in the grated zucchini.
- Slowly add the dry ingredients to the wet ingredients, mixing just until combined.
- Fold in the chocolate chips.

- Spoon the batter into the prepared muffin cups, filling each about 2/3 full.
- Bake the muffins for 20-25 minutes or until a toothpick inserted into the center comes out clean.
- Remove the muffins from the oven and let them cool in the pan for 5 minutes before transferring to a wire rack to cool completely.

These chocolate zucchini muffins are a great way to use up zucchini and it's perfect for a snack or breakfast. They are moist and *chocolatey*, and the zucchini provides added moisture and makes them a little healthier. You can also add nuts or dried fruits to the batter if desired.

<u>BREAKFAST BERRY CRISP</u>

Here's a recipe for Breakfast Berry Crisp:

Ingredients:

- 4 cups mixed berries (such as blueberries, raspberries, blackberries and strawberries)
- 1/4 cup granulated sugar
- 2 tablespoons cornstarch
- 1 teaspoon lemon juice
- 1/2 cup rolled oats
- 1/4 cup all-purpose flour
- 1/4 cup brown sugar
- 1/4 teaspoon ground cinnamon
- 1/4 cup unsalted butter, chilled and diced
- 1/4 cup chopped nuts (such as almonds or pecans) (optional)

Directions:

- Preheat your oven to 375°F.
- In a mixing bowl, combine the mixed berries, sugar, cornstarch, and lemon juice. Pour the mixture into an 8x8 inch baking dish.
- In another mixing bowl, combine the oats, flour, brown sugar, cinnamon, butter, and nuts (if using). Mix until crumbly.
- Sprinkle the oat mixture over the berries in the baking dish.

- Bake in the preheated oven for 30-35 minutes, or until the topping is golden brown and the berry filling is bubbly.
- Let the crisp cool for a few minutes before serving. It can be served warm or at room temperature.

This breakfast berry crisp is perfect for a weekend brunch or a healthy breakfast. The combination of different berries and the crisp oat topping make it a delicious and nutritious way to start your day. You can also use frozen berries if you don't have fresh ones and you can add some yogurt or ice cream on top for a more decadent treat.

<u>GOLDEN OVERNIGHT OAT WITH ORANGE FLAVOR</u>

Here's a recipe for Golden Overnight Oats with Orange Flavor:

Ingredients:

- 1 cup rolled oats
- 1 cup milk (dairy or non-dairy)
- 1/2 cup plain Greek yogurt
- 1/4 cup honey
- 1 tablespoon chia seeds
- 1 teaspoon vanilla extract
- 1 teaspoon grated orange zest
- 1/4 cup fresh orange juice
- Toppings such as chopped nuts, dried fruit, shredded coconut (optional)

Directions:

- In a mixing bowl, combine the oats, milk, yogurt, honey, chia seeds, vanilla extract, orange zest, and orange juice.
- Mix well and transfer the mixture to a sealable container or mason jar.
- Refrigerate overnight or for at least 4 hours to allow the oats to absorb the liquid and soften.
- Before serving, give the oats a good stir and adjust the sweetness or consistency with additional honey or milk, if needed.
- Serve the oats cold and add toppings of your choice, such as chopped nuts, dried fruit, or shredded coconut.

This recipe is a delicious and healthy way to start your day. The combination of orange flavor with the oats and yogurt make it a tasty and nutritious breakfast. Oats are a great source of fiber, protein and they help keep you full for a long time. The orange juice and zest add a fresh citrusy flavor and a boost of vitamin C. And you can top with your favorite fresh fruits, nuts, or seeds for an extra crunch.

<u>BLUEBERRY PANCAKES WITH OATMEAL</u>

Here's a recipe for Blueberry Pancakes:

Ingredients:

- 1 1/2 cups all-purpose flour
- 2 tablespoons sugar
- 2 teaspoons baking powder
- 1/2 teaspoon baking soda
- 1/2 teaspoon salt
- 1 cup milk (dairy or non-dairy)
- 1 egg
- 2 tablespoons unsalted butter, melted
- 1 teaspoon vanilla extract
- 1 cup fresh blueberries
- butter, for cooking
- Maple syrup, for serving

Directions:

- In a mixing bowl, combine the flour, sugar, baking powder, baking soda, and salt.
- In another mixing bowl, whisk together the milk, egg, melted butter, and vanilla extract.
- Pour the mixture of wet ingredients into the dry ingredients and mix until it is evenly combined. Then gently fold in the blueberries.
- Heat a griddle or a large skillet over medium heat. Grease the surface by melting a small amount of butter on it.

- Using a ladle or measuring cup, pour the batter onto the griddle. Cook the pancakes for 2-3 minutes or until bubbles form on the surface, then flip and cook for an additional 1-2 minutes on the other side.
- Serve the pancakes warm with butter and maple syrup.

These blueberry pancakes are a delicious and classic breakfast treat. The fresh blueberries add a burst of flavor and a pop of color to the pancakes. You can also use frozen blueberries if you don't have fresh ones, just be careful not to overmix the batter or the blueberries might turn the pancakes purple. These pancakes can be enjoyed with butter and maple syrup or with whipped cream and fresh berries.

GREEN PEANUT BUTTER-BANANA SMOOTHIE

Here's a recipe for a Green Peanut Butter-Banana Smoothie:

Ingredients:

- 1 ripe banana
- 1 cup fresh spinach or kale leaves
- 2 tablespoons of creamy peanut butter
- 1/2 cup plain Greek yogurt
- 1/4 cup of unsweetened almond milk
- 1 tablespoon honey (or to taste)
- 1/2 teaspoon vanilla extract
- 1/2 cup ice

Directions:

- Peel the banana and cut it into chunks, then place it in the freezer for at least 2 hours.
- In a blender, combine the frozen banana, spinach or kale, yogurt, almond milk, peanut butter, honey, vanilla extract, and ice.
- Blend on high speed until it is smooth and creamy, about 1-2 minutes.
- Pour the smoothie into a glass and serve immediately.

This green peanut butter-banana smoothie is a delicious and healthy way to start your day or enjoy as a snack. The banana and peanut butter provide a creamy texture and a natural sweetness, while the spinach or kale adds a boost of vitamins and minerals. You can also add other ingredients like chia seeds, flax seeds, or protein powder for extra nutrients, or switch out almond milk for any kind of milk or milk alternatives that you like.

MEDITERRANEAN EGGPLANT SHAKSHUKA

Here's a recipe for Mediterranean Eggplant Shakshuka:

Ingredients:

- 2 tablespoons olive oil
- 1 medium onion, diced
- 2 cloves garlic, minced
- 1 medium eggplant, diced
- 1 red bell pepper, diced
- 1 teaspoon ground cumin
- 1/2 teaspoon smoked paprika
- 1/4 teaspoon cayenne pepper
- 1 can (14.5 oz) diced tomatoes
- Salt and pepper
- 4 eggs
- Fresh parsley or cilantro, for serving
- Feta cheese, for serving
- Pita bread or crusty bread, for serving

Directions:

- In a large skillet, heat the olive oil over medium heat. Add the onion and garlic and cook for about 3-4 minutes or until softened.
- Add the eggplant and red bell pepper to the skillet and continue to cook for about 5 minutes or until the vegetables are tender.
- Stir in the cumin, smoked paprika, cayenne pepper, diced tomatoes, salt, and pepper.

- Bring the mixture to a simmer and let it cook for 10-15 minutes or until the tomatoes have thickened and the vegetables are very tender.
- Using the back of a spoon, make four wells in the tomato mixture. Crack an egg into each well.
- Cover the skillet and cook the eggs for about 3-5 minutes or until the whites are set but the yolks are still runny.
- Serve the shakshuka hot with fresh parsley or cilantro, crumbled feta cheese, and pita bread or crusty bread on the side.

This Mediterranean Eggplant Shakshuka is a delicious and healthy dish that is perfect for brunch or breakfast. The combination of eggplant, bell pepper and tomatoes with the spices and eggs make this dish a hearty and flavorful meal that is easy to make. You can also add some chickpeas or other vegetables to make it more filling. It's a great way to use up eggplants and it's gluten-free and can be enjoyed as a vegetarian dish or you can add some ground meat or sausage to make it more protein-packed.

<u>FRITTATAS WITH SPINACH AND RED PEPPERS</u>

Here's a recipe for Spinach and Red Pepper Frittatas:

Ingredients:
- 8 eggs
- 1/4 cup heavy cream or milk
- Salt and pepper
- 1 tablespoon olive oil
- 1/2 red pepper, diced
- 1/2 onion, diced
- 2 cloves garlic, minced
- 2 cups fresh spinach
- 1/4 cup grated Parmesan cheese
- 2 tablespoons chopped fresh parsley (optional)

Directions:

- Preheat your oven to 350°F.
- In a mixing bowl, whisk together the eggs, cream or milk, salt, and pepper.
- In a skillet, heat olive oil over medium heat. Add the diced red pepper, onion, and garlic. Cook for about 3-4 minutes or until softened.
- Add the spinach to the skillet and cook for about 2-3 minutes or until wilted.
- Pour the egg mixture over the vegetables in the skillet and cook over medium heat until the edges start to set, about 2-3 minutes.

- Sprinkle the grated Parmesan cheese over the frittata and transfer the skillet to the preheated oven.
- Bake the frittata for about 8-10 minutes or until the center is set and the top is golden brown.
- Remove the skillet from the oven and let the frittata cool for a few minutes before slicing.
- Garnish with chopped parsley, if desired and serve warm.

This spinach and red pepper frittata is a great way to use up fresh vegetables and it's perfect for brunch or breakfast. It's a great source of protein and healthy fats. You can also add other vegetables or cheese to make it more flavorful. And you can adjust the seasoning to your liking and add some herbs or spices if you want.

<u>AVOCADO-EGG SALAD TOAST</u>

Here's a recipe for Avocado-Egg Salad Toast:

Ingredients:

- 4 hard-boiled eggs
- 1 ripe avocado
- 1/4 cup mayonnaise
- 2 tablespoons chopped fresh chives
- 1 tablespoon Dijon mustard
- Salt and pepper
- 4 slices of bread, toasted

Directions:

- Peel and mash the hard-boiled eggs in a mixing bowl.
- Cut open the avocado in half, remove the pit and scoop out the flesh. Mash the avocado in a separate bowl.
- Add the mashed avocado to the eggs and mix well.
- Stir in the mayonnaise, chives, and Dijon mustard. Season with salt and pepper to taste.
- Spread the egg salad on top of the toasted bread slices.
- Serve immediately and Enjoy!

This avocado-egg salad toast is a delicious and easy to make breakfast or lunch dish. It's a great way to use up hard-boiled eggs and it's a healthy and tasty option. The avocado adds a creamy texture and flavor to the egg salad and it makes it more nutritious. You can add other ingredients like bacon, cheese or herbs to make it more flavorful. You can also use whole wheat bread, or any kind of bread you like to make it healthier.

CHAPTER FOUR

Lunch

CHICKEN LETTUCE WRAPS

Here's a recipe for Chicken Lettuce Wraps:

Ingredients:

- 1 pound ground chicken
- 1 tablespoon vegetable oil
- 1 small onion, diced
- 2 cloves garlic, minced
- 1 red bell pepper, diced
- 2 tablespoons hoisin sauce
- 2 tablespoons soy sauce
- 2 teaspoons rice vinegar
- 1 teaspoon sesame oil
- Salt and pepper
- 1 head of butter lettuce or bibb lettuce
- Toppings such as diced green onions, chopped cilantro, diced red bell pepper and diced avocado

Directions:

- In a large skillet, heat the vegetable oil over medium-high heat. Add the ground chicken and cook until browned, about 5-7 minutes.
- Add the onion, garlic, and red bell pepper to the skillet and continue to cook for another 3-5 minutes or until the vegetables are softened.

- Stir in the hoisin sauce, rice vinegar, soy sauce, and sesame oil and season with pepper and salt to taste.
- Cook for an additional 2-3 minutes, or until the sauce has thickened and the chicken is cooked through.
- Put out the heat on the skillet and let it cool for a few minutes.
- Arrange the lettuce leaves on a plate.
- Using a slotted spoon, spoon the chicken mixture into the center of each lettuce leaf.
- Top with desired toppings such as diced green onions, chopped cilantro, diced red bell pepper and diced avocado,
- Fold the lettuce leaf around the filling and enjoy!

This chicken lettuce wraps recipe is a delicious and healthy way to enjoy a meal. The combination of ground chicken and vegetables with the hoisin sauce, soy sauce, and rice vinegar make it a flavorful and satisfying dish. The lettuce leaves provide a crispy and refreshing contrast to the filling and it makes it a low-carb and low-calorie option. You can also add some peanuts or cashews for an extra crunch and use any kind of lettuce you prefer.

<u>BEEF SKEWERS</u>

Here's a recipe for Beef Skewers:

Ingredients:

- 1 lb beef sirloin or flank steak, cut into 1-inch cubes
- 1/4 cup soy sauce
- 2 tablespoons brown sugar
- 2 cloves garlic, minced
- 1 tablespoon vegetable oil
- 1 teaspoon ground ginger
- 1/4 teaspoon black pepper
- Bamboo skewers (soaked in water for at least 30 minutes)
- Salt to taste
- Optional: vegetables like bell peppers, onions, mushrooms to alternate with beef cubes on skewers

Directions:

- In a mixing bowl, whisk together the soy sauce, brown sugar, garlic, vegetable oil, ginger, and pepper. Add the beef cubes to the marinade, toss to coat, and let it marinate in the refrigerator for at least 30 minutes or up to 2 hours.
- Preheat your grill to about medium-high heat.
- Remove the beef cubes from the marinade, discarding the remaining marinade. Thread the beef cubes onto the soaked skewers, alternating with vegetables if using.
- Season the skewers with salt to taste.

- Grill the skewers for 8-10 minutes or until the beef is cooked to your desired level of doneness, turning occasionally.
- Remove the skewers from the grill and let them rest for a few minutes before serving.

These beef skewers are a delicious and easy way to enjoy a meal. The marinade provides a great flavor to the beef and the skewers make it easy to cook and serve. You can also use any kind of beef cut you prefer or add any vegetables you like. You can serve it with a side of rice or a salad, or even wrap it in a pita or a tortilla for a sandwich.

<u>ROASTED PUMPKIN CURRY</u>

Here is a recipe for a roasted pumpkin curry:

Ingredients:

- 1 large pumpkin, peeled, seeded and cut into 1-inch cubes
- 1 tablespoon olive oil
- Salt and pepper, to taste
- 1 onion, diced
- 2 cloves of garlic, minced
- 1 tablespoon ginger, grated
- 2 tablespoons curry powder
- 1 can of coconut milk
- 1 cup of vegetable broth
- 1 teaspoon sugar
- 1 teaspoon cumin powder
- 1 teaspoon coriander powder
- 1/2 teaspoon turmeric powder
- 1/2 teaspoon cayenne pepper (optional)
- 1/4 cup chopped fresh cilantro, for garnish

Directions:

- Preheat the oven to 400°F.
- Toss the pumpkin with olive oil, salt and pepper and spread on a baking sheet. Roast for 25-30 minutes or until tender.
- In a large pot or Dutch oven, heat some oil and sauté the onion, garlic and ginger until softened.
- Stir in the curry powder and cook for about a minute.

- Add the roasted pumpkin, coconut milk, vegetable broth, sugar, cumin, coriander, turmeric and cayenne pepper. Bring to a boil, then reduce the heat and simmer for 20 minutes.
- Taste and adjust the seasoning as you desire.
- Serve over rice or with naan bread and garnish with cilantro.

Note: You can also use other vegetables like carrots, bell peppers, or cauliflower, along with pumpkin for variation.

<u>SHRIMP MAPLE SKEWERS</u>

Ingredients:

- 1 pound large shrimp, peeled and deveined
- 1/4 cup pure maple syrup
- 2 tablespoons olive oil
- 2 cloves of garlic, minced
- 1 teaspoon smoked paprika
- 1/2 teaspoon salt
- 1/4 teaspoon black pepper

Directions:

- In a small bowl, mix together the maple syrup, olive oil, garlic, smoked paprika, salt, and pepper.
- Thread the shrimp onto skewers and brush them with the maple syrup mixture.
- Preheat your grill or grill pan to high heat. Grill the skewers for 2-3 minutes per side, or until the shrimp is pink and cooked through.
- Serve with a side of your choice or with a salad

PAN-SEARED SCALLOPS

Ingredients:

- 1 pound scallops, rinsed and patted dry
- 2 tablespoons butter
- 2 tablespoons olive oil
- Salt and pepper, to taste
- 1 lemon, cut into wedges

Directions:

- Season the scallops with pepper and salt.
- In a large skillet, heat the butter and olive oil over medium-high heat until the butter is melted.
- Add the scallops to the skillet and cook for 2-3 minutes per side, or until golden brown and cooked through.
- Serve with a squeeze of lemon juice and a sprinkle of salt.

<u>SHRIMP TOMATO SALAD</u>

Ingredients:

- 1 pound of cooked shrimp, peeled and deveined
- 2 cups cherry tomatoes, halved
- 1/4 cup chopped fresh basil
- 2 cloves of garlic, minced
- 2 tablespoons olive oil
- 1 tablespoon red wine vinegar
- Salt and pepper, to taste

Directions:

- In a large bowl, combine the shrimp, tomatoes, basil, and garlic.
- In a small bowl, whisk together the olive oil and red wine vinegar.
- Drizzle the dressing over the shrimp and tomato mixture and toss to combine.
- Season with pepper and salt to taste.
- Serve chilled or at room temperature as a side dish or an appetizer.

TOMATO SALMON BOWL

Ingredients:

- 4 (6-ounce) salmon fillets
- Salt and pepper, to taste
- 2 tablespoons olive oil
- 1 pint cherry tomatoes, halved
- 1/4 cup chopped fresh basil
- 1/4 cup chopped fresh parsley
- 2 cloves of garlic, minced
- 2 tablespoons red wine vinegar
- 1/2 cup quinoa or brown rice

Directions:

- Season the salmon fillets with salt and pepper.
- In a large skillet, heat the olive oil over medium-high heat.
- Add the salmon fillets to the skillet and cook for 3-4 minutes per side or until cooked through.
- In a separate pan, cook the quinoa or brown rice according to package directions.
- In a large bowl, combine the cherry tomatoes, basil, parsley, garlic, and red wine vinegar.
- Place the cooked quinoa or brown rice in a bowl and top with the cooked salmon and tomato mixture.

<u>GROUND CHICKEN WITH TOMATOES</u>

Ingredients:

- 1 pound ground chicken
- 1 onion, diced
- 2 cloves of garlic, minced
- 1 pint cherry tomatoes, halved
- 1 teaspoon paprika
- 1/2 teaspoon cumin powder
- 1/2 teaspoon salt
- 1/4 teaspoon black pepper
- 2 tablespoons olive oil
- 1/4 cup chopped fresh parsley

Directions:

- Heat the olive oil in a large skillet over medium-high heat.
- Add the garlic, onion and sauté until softened.
- Add the ground chicken to the skillet and cook until browned.
- Stir in the paprika, cherry tomatoes, salt, cumin, and pepper.
- Cook for an additional 5-7 minutes, or until the tomatoes are soft.
- Stir in the chopped parsley.
- Serve over rice, pasta or quinoa.

BEEF AND VEGGIE BURGERS

Ingredients:

- 1 pound ground beef
- 1/2 cup grated carrots
- 1/2 cup grated zucchini
- 1/4 cup breadcrumbs
- 1 egg, lightly beaten
- 2 cloves of garlic, minced
- 1 teaspoon salt
- 1/4 teaspoon black pepper
- Olive oil, for cooking
- Buns and toppings of your choice

Directions:

- In a large bowl, combine the ground beef, grated carrots, grated zucchini, breadcrumbs, egg, garlic, salt, and pepper.
- Mix until well combined.
- Divide the mixture into 4-6 portions and shape into patties.
- In a skillet or grill, heat some olive oil over medium-high heat.
- Add the patties to the skillet or grill and cook for 4-5 minutes per side or until cooked through.
- Serve on buns with the toppings of your choice.

EGGS AND AVOCADO ENDIVE WRAPS

Ingredients:

- 4 large eggs
- 2 ripe avocados
- 1/4 teaspoon salt
- 1/4 teaspoon black pepper
- 4 heads of endive leaves
- 1/4 cup chopped fresh cilantro
- 1/4 cup chopped fresh chives

Directions:

- Bring a pot of water to a boil and gently lower the eggs into the water. Cook for 8-10 minutes.
- Remove the eggs after they are done and place them in a bowl of ice water.
- When the eggs are cool, peel and chop them.
- Cut the avocados in half, remove the seed, and scoop the avocado flesh out into a bowl. Mash the avocado with a fork and add the salt and pepper.
- Carefully separate the endive leaves, leaving them attached at the base.
- Spread a spoonful of mashed avocado on each endive leaf, then top with some chopped eggs.
- Sprinkle with chives cilantro.
- Carefully roll up the endive leaves to make wraps.

GREEK CUCUMBER SALAD

Ingredients:

- 1 large English cucumber, sliced
- 1/2 red onion, thinly sliced
- 1/2 cup kalamata olives, pitted
- 1/2 cup crumbled feta cheese
- 1/4 cup chopped fresh dill
- 2 tablespoons red wine vinegar
- 1 tablespoon olive oil
- Salt and pepper, to taste

Directions:

- In a large bowl, combine the cucumber, olives, red onion, dill and feta cheese.
- In a small bowl, whisk together the red wine vinegar, olive oil, salt, and pepper.
- Pour the dressing over the mixture with cucumber and toss to coat.
- Let it sit for at least 30 minutes in the fridge to allow the flavors to meld together.
- Serve chilled.

BEEF AND SPINACH BURGERS

Ingredients:

- 1 pound ground beef
- 1/2 cup chopped spinach
- 1/4 cup breadcrumbs
- 1 egg, lightly beaten
- 2 cloves of garlic, minced
- 1 teaspoon salt
- 1/4 teaspoon black pepper
- Olive oil, for cooking
- Buns and toppings of your choice

Directions:

- In a large bowl, combine the ground beef, chopped spinach, breadcrumbs, egg, garlic, salt, and pepper.
- Mix until well combined.
- Divide the mixture into 4-6 portions and shape into patties.
- In a skillet or grill, heat some olive oil over medium-high heat.
- Add the patties to the skillet or grill and cook for 4-5 minutes per side or until cooked through.
- Serve on buns with toppings of your choice.

Please note that you can adjust the spices, herbs, and quantities as per your taste preference.

<u>EUROPEAN BEET SOUP</u>

Ingredients:

- 2 tablespoons olive oil
- 1 onion, diced
- 2 cloves garlic, minced
- 2 medium beets, peeled and diced
- 3 cups chicken or vegetable broth
- 1 teaspoon caraway seeds
- Salt and pepper, to taste
- Sour cream or yogurt, for garnish (optional)

Directions:

- In a large pot, heat the olive oil over medium heat. Add the onion and garlic and sauté until softened, about 5 minutes.
- Add the beets, broth, caraway seeds, salt, and pepper to the pot. Bring to a boil, then reduce the heat and simmer until the beets are tender, about 20 minutes.
- Use an immersion blender or a regular blender to puree the soup until smooth.
- Taste and adjust the seasoning as required.
- Serve hot, garnished with sour cream or yogurt, if desired.

<u>PASTA WITH ASPARAGUS</u>

Ingredients:

- 8 oz spaghetti or other pasta
- 1 lb asparagus, trimmed and cut into 1-inch pieces
- 2 cloves garlic, minced
- 2 tablespoons olive oil
- Salt and pepper, to taste
- 1/4 cup of grated Parmesan cheese
- 2 tablespoons chopped fresh parsley or basil, for garnish

Directions:

- Bring a large pot of salted water to a boil and cook the pasta according to package directions. Reserve about 1 cup of the pasta cooking water.
- While the pasta cooks, heat the olive oil in a large skillet over medium heat. Add the garlic and asparagus and sauté until the asparagus is tender, about 5 minutes.
- Drain the pasta and add it to the skillet with the asparagus. Toss until well combined.
- If the pasta seems dry, add some of the reserved pasta cooking water to the skillet, a little at a time, until you achieve your desired consistency.
- Season with pepper and salt to taste.
- Serve the pasta in bowls, topped with grated Parmesan cheese and chopped parsley or basil.

<u>TURKEY BURGERS</u>

Ingredients:

- 1 pound ground turkey
- 1/4 cup breadcrumbs
- 1/4 cup grated Parmesan cheese
- 1 egg, lightly beaten
- 2 cloves garlic, minced
- 1/4 cup chopped fresh parsley or cilantro
- Salt and pepper, to taste
- 4 hamburger buns
- Lettuce, tomato, and other toppings, as desired

Directions:

- In a large bowl, mix together the ground turkey, breadcrumbs, Parmesan cheese, egg, garlic, parsley or cilantro, salt and pepper.
- Divide the mixture into 4 equal portions and shape each portion into a patty.
- Heat a large skillet over medium-high heat and cook the patties for about 5 minutes per side, or until cooked through.
- Serve the turkey burgers on hamburger buns with lettuce, tomato, and other toppings of your choice.

PASTA WITH ZUCCHINI AND TOMATOES

Ingredients:

- 8 oz pasta of your choice
- 2 tbsp olive oil
- 1 onion, chopped
- 2 cloves garlic, minced
- 2 zucchinis, sliced
- 1 can (28 oz) diced tomatoes
- Salt and pepper, to taste
- Fresh basil, chopped (optional)
- Grated Parmesan cheese (optional)

Directions:

- Cook the pasta according to the package directions.
- In a separate pan, heat the olive oil over medium heat. Add the onion and garlic and sauté for 2-3 minutes or until softened.
- Add the zucchinis to the pan and sauté for 5-7 minutes or until they are tender.
- Stir in the diced tomatoes and bring to a simmer. Season with pepper and salt to taste.
- Drain the cooked pasta and add it to the pan with the sauce. Toss to combine.
- Serve with fresh basil and grated Parmesan cheese, if desired.

BEEF AND MOZZARELLA BURGERS

Ingredients:

- 1 lb ground beef
- 1/4 cup grated mozzarella cheese
- 1/4 cup breadcrumbs
- 1 egg
- 1 tbsp Worcestershire sauce
- 1 tsp garlic powder
- Salt and pepper, to taste
- 4 hamburger buns
- Lettuce, tomato, and condiments of your choice

Directions:

- In a large bowl, combine the ground beef, mozzarella cheese, breadcrumbs, egg, Worcestershire sauce, garlic powder, salt and pepper. Mix well.
- Form the mixture into 4 patties.
- Preheat a grill or grill pan to medium-high heat. Grill the patties for 3-4 minutes per side or until fully cooked.
- Toast the hamburger buns if desired
- Assemble the burgers with lettuce, tomato and condiments of your choice.

TUNA STUFFED AVOCADO

Ingredients:

- 2 ripe avocados
- 2 cans of tuna, drained
- 2 tbsp mayonnaise
- 2 tbsp chopped onion
- 2 tbsp chopped cilantro
- 2 tbsp lime juice
- Salt and pepper, to taste

Directions:

- Cut the avocados in half and remove the pit.
- In a mixing bowl, combine the tuna, mayonnaise, onion, cilantro, lime juice, salt and pepper.
- Stuff the mixture into the avocado halves.
- Serve chilled.

SHRIMP LETTUCE WRAPS

Ingredients:

- 1 lb large shrimp, peeled and deveined
- 1 tbsp olive oil
- 1 tbsp sesame oil
- 2 cloves garlic, minced
- 1 tsp ginger, grated
- 1/2 cup hoisin sauce
- 1/4 cup soy sauce
- 2 tbsp rice vinegar
- 2 tbsp brown sugar
- 1 head of butter lettuce, with the leaves separated
- 1/4 cup green onions, thinly sliced
- 1/4 cup cilantro, chopped

Directions:

- Over medium-high heat, heat a large skillet. Add the olive oil, sesame oil, garlic, and ginger. Sauté for about 1-2 minutes or until it is fragrant.
- Add the shrimp to the pan and cook for 2-3 minutes per side or until pink and cooked through.
- In a small bowl, mix together the hoisin sauce, soy sauce, rice vinegar, and brown sugar.
- Add the sauce to the pan with the shrimp and stir to coat.
- Serve the shrimp mixture in the lettuce cups, topped with green onions and cilantro.

<u>LEMONY SCALLOPS</u>

Ingredients:

- 1 lb sea scallops
- Salt and pepper, to taste
- 2 tbsp olive oil
- 1 tbsp butter
- 2 cloves garlic, minced
- 1/4 cup dry white wine
- 1/4 cup chicken broth
- 2 tbsp lemon juice
- 2 tbsp chopped parsley

Directions:

- Season the scallops with pepper and salt.
- Heat a skillet over high heat. Add the olive oil and butter.
- Once the butter is melted, add the scallops and cook for 2-3 minutes per side or until golden brown.
- Remove the scallops from the pan and set them aside.
- Reduce the heat of the pan to medium. Add the garlic and sauté for about 30 seconds.
- Pour in the white wine and chicken broth, and bring to a simmer.
- Stir in the lemon juice and parsley, and cook for 1-2 minutes or until the sauce is slightly thickened.
- Return the scallops to the pan and toss to coat with the sauce.

- Serve immediately, garnished with additional parsley if desired.

CHAPTER FIVE

Dinner

STUFFED ZUCCHINI BOATS

Ingredients:

- 4 medium zucchinis
- 1 tbsp olive oil
- 1 onion, diced
- 2 cloves garlic, minced
- 1 lb ground beef or turkey
- 1 can (14.5 oz) diced tomatoes
- 1/4 cup grated Parmesan cheese
- 1/4 cup breadcrumbs
- Salt and pepper, to taste
- 1 cup of shredded mozzarella cheese

Directions:

- Preheat the oven to 375 F (190 C).
- Cut the zucchinis in half lengthwise and scoop out the seeds with a spoon.
- Heat the olive oil in a pan over medium heat. Add the onion and garlic, and sauté for 2-3 minutes or until softened.
- Add the ground beef or turkey and cook until browned. Drain any excess fat.

- Stir in the diced tomatoes, Parmesan cheese, breadcrumbs, salt and pepper.
- Spoon the mixture into the zucchini boats and top with shredded mozzarella cheese.
- Place the zucchini boats on a baking sheet and bake for 25-30 minutes or until the zucchinis are tender and the cheese is golden and bubbly.

CHICKEN CUTLETS

Ingredients:

- 4 boneless, skinless chicken breasts
- 1/2 cup flour
- 2 eggs, beaten
- 1 cup breadcrumbs
- 1/4 cup grated Parmesan cheese
- Salt and pepper, to taste
- 2 tbsp olive oil

Directions:

- Place the chicken breasts between two sheets of plastic wrap and pound until they are about 1/4 inch thickness.
- Place the flour, breadcrumbs and eggs in separate shallow dishes. Mix Parmesan cheese, salt and pepper into the breadcrumbs.
- Dredge the chicken in the flour. Shake off any excess flour. Dip the chicken in the eggs and then coat in the breadcrumb mixture.
- Heat the olive oil in a pan over medium-high heat. Add the chicken and cook for 2-3 minutes per side or until golden brown and cooked through.

<u>HALIBUT CURRY</u>

Ingredients:

- 1 lb halibut or other white fish fillets
- 1 tbsp olive oil
- 1 onion, diced
- 2 cloves garlic, minced
- 1 tbsp curry powder
- 1 can (14.5 oz) diced tomatoes
- 1 cup coconut milk
- Salt and pepper, to taste
- Fresh cilantro, chopped (optional)

Directions:

- Cut the halibut or other white fish fillets into bite-sized pieces.
- In a pan, heat the olive oil over medium heat. Add the onion and garlic, and sauté for 2-3 minutes or until softened.
- Stir in the curry powder and cook for an additional 1-2 minutes.
- Stir in the diced tomatoes and coconut milk. Bring to a simmer.
- Add the halibut or other white fish fillets to the pan, and cook for 3-4 minutes or until the fish is cooked through.
- Season with pepper and salt to taste.
- Serve over rice and garnish with fresh cilantro if desired.

<u>ROSEMARY CHICKEN</u>

Ingredients:

- 4 boneless, skinless chicken breasts
- 2 tbsp olive oil
- 2 cloves garlic, minced
- 2 tbsp fresh rosemary, chopped
- Salt and pepper, to taste
- Lemon wedges for serving

Directions:

- Season the chicken breasts with pepper and salt.
- Heat your skillet over medium-high heat. Add the olive oil and garlic. Sauté for 1-2 minutes or until fragrant.
- Add the chicken breasts to the skillet, and cook for 3-4 minutes per side or until golden brown and cooked through.
- Remove and set aside the chicken from the skillet.
- In the same skillet, add the fresh rosemary, sauté for 1-2 minutes or until fragrant.
- Return the chicken to the skillet and toss to coat in the rosemary mixture.
- Serve with lemon wedges.

<u>LEMONY SALMON</u>

Ingredients:

- 4 salmon fillets
- Salt and pepper, to taste
- 2 tbsp olive oil
- 2 tbsp lemon juice
- 1 tsp Dijon mustard
- 1 tsp honey
- 1 clove garlic, minced
- 1 tbsp chopped parsley

Directions:

- Season the salmon fillets with pepper and salt.
- In a small bowl, mix together the olive oil, lemon juice, Dijon mustard, honey, and garlic.
- Heat a skillet over medium-high heat. Add the salmon fillets, skin side down.
- Brush the top of the fillets with the lemon mixture.
- Cook the salmon for 3-4 minutes per side, or until the fish is cooked through and the skin is crispy.
- Remove the salmon from the skillet and sprinkle with chopped parsley.

<u>HERB SALMON</u>

Ingredients:

- 4 salmon fillets
- Salt and pepper, to taste
- 2 tbsp olive oil
- 2 tbsp chopped fresh herbs (such as parsley, dill, thyme, and basil)
- 1 tbsp lemon juice
- 1 clove garlic, minced

Directions:

- Season the salmon fillets with pepper and salt.
- In a small bowl, mix together the herbs, olive oil, garlic and lemon juice.
- Heat your skillet over medium-high heat. Add the salmon fillets, skin side down.
- Brush the top of the fillets with the herb mixture.
- Cook the salmon for about 3-4 minutes per side, or until the fish is cooked through and the skin becomes crispy.

CANTALOUPE GNOCCHI

Ingredients:

- 1 cantaloupe, peeled and seeded
- 1 cup all-purpose flour
- 1 egg
- 1/4 cup grated Parmesan cheese
- Salt and pepper, to taste

Directions:

- In a food processor, puree the cantaloupe until smooth.
- In a large mixing bowl, combine the cantaloupe puree, flour, egg, Parmesan cheese, salt, and pepper. Mix until a dough forms.
- On a floured surface, roll the dough into long, thin ropes. Cut the ropes into small, bite-sized pieces.
- Bring a large pot of salted water to a boiler. Add the gnocchi and cook for 2-3 minutes, or until they float to the surface.
- Drain the gnocchi and serve with your favorite sauce.

<u>VEGGIE RISOTTO</u>

Ingredients:

- 1 tbsp olive oil
- 1 small onion, diced
- 2 cloves garlic, minced
- 1 cup Arborio rice
- 3 cups vegetable broth
- 1 cup diced mixed vegetables (such as carrots, peas, and bell peppers)
- 1/4 cup grated Parmesan cheese
- Salt and pepper, to taste

Directions:

- In a large saucepan, heat the olive oil over medium heat. Add the onion and garlic and sauté for 2-3 minutes, or until softened.
- Add the Arborio rice and stir to coat with the oil.
- Slowly pour in the vegetable broth, one ladleful at a time, stirring constantly. Allow the liquid to be absorbed before adding the next ladleful.
- Once all of the broth has been added and the rice is cooked through, stir in the diced vegetables.
- Remove the pan from the heat and stir in the Parmesan cheese. Season with salt and pepper to taste.
- Serve and enjoy!

LEMON PEPPER TURKEY

Ingredients:

- 1 turkey breast
- 1/4 cup olive oil
- 2 tbsp lemon juice
- 1 tsp lemon zest
- 1 tsp black pepper
- Salt, to taste

Directions:

- Preheat your oven to 350°F (175°C).
- In a small bowl, mix together the olive oil, lemon juice, lemon zest, black pepper, and salt.
- Place the turkey breast in a roasting pan and brush the lemon pepper mixture over the turkey.
- Roast the turkey for about 1 hour and 15 minutes or until the internal temperature reaches 165°F (74°C).
- Let the turkey rest for 10-15 minutes before slicing and serving.
- Please note that cook time and serving sizes may vary depending on your oven and the size of the turkey breast.

<u>CHICKEN PICCATA</u>

Ingredients:

- 4 boneless, skinless chicken breasts
- Salt and pepper, to taste
- 1/2 cup all-purpose flour
- 1/4 cup olive oil
- 1/4 cup butter
- 1/2 cup chicken broth
- 1/2 cup freshly squeezed lemon juice
- 2 cloves garlic, minced
- 2 tbsp capers
- 1/4 cup chopped fresh parsley

Directions:

- Season the chicken breasts with salt and pepper, and then dust them with flour.
- Heat the butter and olive oil in a large skillet over medium-high heat.
- Add the chicken breasts and cook for 3-4 minutes per side, or until golden brown and cooked through.
- Remove and set aside the chicken from the skillet.
- In the same skillet, add the chicken broth, lemon juice, garlic, capers, and parsley. Bring the mixture to a boil, and then reduce the heat and let it simmer for 2-3 minutes.
- Return the chicken to the skillet and spoon the sauce over the chicken.
- Serve and enjoy!

<u>WHOLE ROASTED TROUT</u>

Ingredients:

- 1 whole trout, cleaned and scaled
- Salt and pepper, to taste
- 2 cloves of garlic, thinly sliced
- 2 lemon slices
- 1 tbsp olive oil
- 1 tbsp butter
- 2 sprigs of fresh thyme

Directions:

- Preheat your oven to 425°F (220°C)
- Season the outside and inside of the trout with pepper and salt.
- Stuff the trout with the garlic, lemon slices, and thyme.
- Place the trout on a baking sheet that is lined with foil and brush with olive oil and butter.
- Roast the trout in the oven for 15-20 minutes, or until the flesh is cooked through and the skin is crispy.
- Remove the trout from the oven and let it rest for a few minutes before serving.

<u>TURKEY AND KALE SAUTÉ</u>

Ingredients:

- 1 lb ground turkey
- 2 cloves of garlic, minced
- 1 onion, diced
- 1 bunch of kale, washed and chopped
- 2 tbsp olive oil
- Salt and pepper, to taste
- 1/4 cup of grated Parmesan cheese

Directions:

- In a large skillet over medium-high heat, sauté the ground turkey, garlic, and onion in olive oil until the turkey is browned and cooked through.
- Season with salt and pepper.
- Add the kale to the skillet and sauté until it is wilted and tender.
- Remove the skillet from the heat and stir in the Parmesan cheese.
- Serve and enjoy!

Please note that cook time may vary depending on the size of your trout.

WINTER APPLE POKE BOWL

Ingredients:

- 1 cup sushi rice
- 2 cups water
- 1 tbsp rice vinegar
- 1 tsp sugar
- 1 tsp salt
- 1/2 cup diced red apple
- 1/2 cup diced green apple
- 1 tbsp soy sauce
- 1 tbsp sesame oil
- 1 tbsp honey
- 1 tsp grated ginger
- 1/4 cup diced green onions
- 1/4 cup sesame seeds

Directions:

- Rinse the rice in a fine mesh strainer under running water until the water runs clear.
- In a medium saucepan, bring the water to a boil. Add the rinsed rice, reduce the heat to low, cover and simmer for 18-20 minutes or until the water is absorbed and the rice is tender.
- In a small bowl mix together the rice vinegar, sugar and salt. Once the rice is cooked, remove it from the heat and add the vinegar mixture. Stir gently and let the rice cool.

- In a medium bowl, whisk together the soy sauce, sesame oil, honey, and ginger. Add the diced apples and toss to coat.
- To serve, divide the rice into bowls and top with the apple mixture, green onions and sesame seeds.

PRAWN AND TOMATO SPAGHETTI

Ingredients:

- 1 lb spaghetti
- 1/4 cup olive oil
- 3 cloves of garlic, minced
- 1 lb prawns, peeled and deveined
- 1 cup cherry tomatoes, halved
- 1/4 cup white wine
- 1/4 cup chopped fresh parsley
- Salt and pepper, to taste

Directions:

- Cook the spaghetti according to the package directions. Drain and set aside.
- In a large skillet over medium heat, heat the olive oil and sauté the garlic for 1-2 minutes or until fragrant.
- Add the prawns and cook until they are pink and cooked through.
- Add the cherry tomatoes and white wine to the skillet and bring to a simmer. Cook for 2-3 minutes or until the tomatoes are tender.
- Toss the spaghetti with the prawn and tomato mixture and parsley. Season with pepper and salt to taste.
- Serve and enjoy!

<u>CHICKEN CACCIATORE</u>

Ingredients:

- 4 chicken thighs
- Salt and pepper, to taste
- 1/4 cup flour
- 1/4 cup olive oil
- 1 onion, diced
- 2 cloves of garlic, minced
- 1 cup sliced mushrooms
- 1 can (14.5 oz) diced tomatoes
- 1/2 cup chicken broth
- 1 tsp dried basil
- 1 tsp dried oregano
- 1/4 cup chopped fresh parsley

Directions:

- Season the chicken thighs with salt and pepper, then dust them with flour.
- In a large skillet over medium-high heat, heat the olive oil and brown the chicken on both sides. Remove and set aside the chicken from the skillet.
- In the same skillet, sauté the onion and garlic until softened.
- Add the mushrooms and sauté for an additional 2-3 minutes or until the mushrooms are tender.
- Stir in the diced tomatoes, chicken broth, basil, and oregano.

- Return the chicken to the skillet and spoon the sauce over it.
- Reduce the heat to low, cover and simmer for 20-25 minutes or until the chicken is cooked through.
- Remove the skillet from the heat and stir in the chopped parsley.
- Serve over pasta or rice.

<u>PEACH STEW</u>

Ingredients:

- 6 ripe peaches, peeled and sliced
- 1/2 cup granulated sugar
- 1 tablespoon cornstarch
- 1 teaspoon ground cinnamon
- 1/4 teaspoon ground nutmeg
- 1/4 teaspoon salt
- 1/4 cup water

Directions:

- In a large pot or Dutch oven, combine the peaches, sugar, cornstarch, cinnamon, nutmeg, and salt. Stir well to combine.
- Add the water and bring the mixture to a boil over medium-high heat.
- Reduce the heat to low and simmer the stew for 20-25 minutes, or until the peaches are tender and the sauce has thickened.
- Serve the stew warm or cold, as desired.

SHRIMP AND SALMON TOMATO STEW

Ingredients:

- -1 lb of shrimp, peeled and deveined
- -1 lb of salmon, cut into chunks
- -1 can of diced tomatoes
- -1 onion, diced
- -2 cloves of garlic, minced
- -1 teaspoon smoked paprika
- -1 teaspoon dried oregano
- -1/4 teaspoon red pepper flakes
- -Salt and pepper, to taste
- -1/4 cup of white wine
- -1 cup of fish or chicken broth
- -1 cup of heavy cream
- -1/4 cup of chopped fresh parsley, for garnish

Directions:

- In a large pot or Dutch oven, heat some oil over medium heat. Add the onion and garlic and sauté until softened and translucent.
- Add the paprika, oregano, and red pepper flakes and sauté for another minute.
- Add the white wine and scrape the bottom of the pot to remove any brown bits.
- Add the diced tomatoes, broth, and cream. Bring the mixture to a simmer.

- Once simmering, add the salmon and shrimp. Cook for about 3-4 minutes or until the shrimp are pink and the salmon is cooked through.
- Season the stew with salt and pepper to taste.
- Serve the stew hot and garnish with fresh parsley.

<u>ZERO-FIBRE CHICKEN DISH</u>

Ingredients:

- 2 boneless, skinless chicken breasts, pounded thin
- salt and pepper
- 1/4 cup of grated Parmesan cheese
- 1/4 cup of heavy cream
- 1/4 cup of chicken broth
- 1 tablespoon of butter
- 1 clove of garlic, minced
- 1 teaspoon of thyme leaves

Directions:

- Season the chicken breasts with pepper and salt.
- Melt the butter in a large skillet over medium-high heat.
- Add the chicken breasts and cook for about 3-4 minutes per side or until golden brown and cooked through.
- Remove the chicken from the skillet and place it on a plate.
- Add the garlic to the skillet and sauté for about 30 seconds.
- Add the chicken broth, cream and thyme leaves. Bring the mixture to a simmer, scraping the bottom of the skillet to remove any brown bits.
- Once the sauce has thickened, add the parmesan cheese. Stir until melted and combined.

- Return the chicken to the skillet and spoon the sauce over the chicken.
- Cook for an additional 2-3 minutes or until the chicken is heated through.
- Serve the chicken with the sauce.

Please note that these recipes are just suggestions, you can adjust them to your taste or dietary restriction.

BRAZILIAN FISH STEW

Ingredients:

- 2 tablespoons olive oil
- 1 onion, finely chopped
- 2 cloves garlic, minced
- 1 red bell pepper, diced
- 1 cup diced tomatoes
- 2 cups fish stock or water
- 1 teaspoon smoked paprika
- 1/2 teaspoon cayenne pepper
- Salt and pepper to taste
- 1 pound white fish fillets, cut into chunks
- 1 cup coconut milk
- Fresh cilantro for garnish

Directions:

- Heat the oil over medium heat in a large pot. Add the onion, garlic, and red bell pepper and sauté until softened.
- Add the tomatoes, fish stock or water, paprika, cayenne, salt and pepper. Bring to a simmer.
- Add the fish and cook until just cooked through, about 5 minutes.
- Stir in the coconut milk and heat through.
- Garnish the fish stew with cilantro and serve with rice.

<u>TURKEY WITH ROSEMARY</u>

Ingredients:

- 1 turkey breast, boneless and skinless
- 2 cloves of garlic, minced
- 2 tablespoons of olive oil
- 2 tablespoons of fresh rosemary leaves
- 1 teaspoon of salt
- 1/2 teaspoon of black pepper
- 1/4 cup of chicken broth
- 1/4 cup of white wine

Directions:

- Preheat the oven to 350°F.
- In a small bowl, mix together the garlic, olive oil, rosemary, salt, and pepper.
- Place the turkey breast in a roasting pan and spread the herb mixture over the turkey.
- Pour the chicken broth and white wine over the turkey.
- Roast the turkey in the oven for about 1 hour, or until the internal temperature reaches 165°F.
- Let the turkey rest for 10 minutes before slicing and serving.

GRILLED SALMON STEAKS

Ingredients:

- 4 salmon steaks
- 2 tablespoons olive oil
- 2 cloves garlic, minced
- 1/4 cup soy sauce
- 2 tablespoons brown sugar
- 2 tablespoons lemon juice
- 1/4 teaspoon black pepper

Directions:

- In a small bowl, mix together the olive oil, garlic, soy sauce, brown sugar, lemon juice, and black pepper.
- Place the salmon steaks in a shallow dish and pour the marinade over them. Let them marinate for at least 30 minutes.
- Preheat grill to high heat.
- Grill the salmon steaks for about 4 minutes per side, or until they are cooked through.
- Serve immediately, garnished with lemon wedges if desired.

FIESTA CHICKEN TACOS

Ingredients:

- 1 pound boneless, skinless chicken breasts
- 1 packet of taco seasoning
- 1/4 cup water
- 8 corn tortillas
- Toppings of your choice (shredded lettuce, diced tomatoes, shredded cheese, sour cream, avocado, etc.)

Directions:

- Cut the chicken breasts into small, bite-sized pieces.
- Over medium heat, heat a large skillet. Add the chicken and cook until browned, about 5 minutes.
- Sprinkle the taco seasoning over the chicken and add the water. Stir properly in order to coat the chicken evenly.
- Cook for an additional 2-3 minutes, or until the chicken is cooked through and the sauce has thickened.
- Heat the tortillas in a skillet or on a griddle until warm and pliable.
- Assemble the tacos by spooning the chicken mixture onto the tortillas and topping with your choice of toppings.

<u>SHRIMP SCAMPI PIZZA</u>

Ingredients:

- 1 pound of pizza dough
- 1/2 cup of butter
- 2 cloves of garlic, minced
- 1/4 teaspoon of red pepper flakes
- 1/4 cup of white wine
- 1 pound of peeled and deveined shrimp
- 1/2 cup of grated Parmesan cheese
- 1/4 cup of chopped parsley
- Salt and pepper to taste

Directions:

- Preheat the oven to 425°F.
- Roll out the pizza dough to your desired thickness and place it on a baking sheet or pizza stone.
- In a pan over medium heat, melt the butter. Add the garlic and red pepper flakes, and sauté for 1-2 minutes.
- Pour in the white wine, and stir in the shrimp. Cook for 2-3 minutes, until the shrimp turn pink.
- Spread the shrimp mixture over the dough, leaving a 1-inch border around the edges.
- Sprinkle the Parmesan cheese over the shrimp, and season with salt and pepper.
- In the preheated oven, bake the pizza for about 12-15 minutes, or until the crust turns golden brown and the cheese is melted.
- Sprinkle with parsley then serve.

CHAPTER SIX

Desserts

VEGAN PECAN TART WITH CHOCOLATE CRUST

Ingredients:

- 1 1/2 cups all-purpose flour
- 1/2 cup cocoa powder
- 1/2 cup sugar
- 1/2 cup vegan butter, chilled and diced
- 1 tsp vanilla extract
- 1/4 tsp salt
- 1 cup pecan halves
- 1/2 cup maple syrup
- 1 tbsp cornstarch
- 1 tsp vanilla extract

Directions:

- In a large mixing bowl, combine the flour, cocoa powder, sugar, and salt. Mix well.
- Add the chilled vegan butter and vanilla extract to the dry ingredients. Mix until the dough comes together and forms a ball.
- Press the dough into a 9-inch tart pan with a removable bottom. Press the dough evenly into the bottom and up the sides of the pan.
- Preheat your oven to 350°F (175°C).

- In a separate mixing bowl, combine the pecan halves, maple syrup, cornstarch, and vanilla extract. Mix well.
- Pour the pecan mixture into the prepared crust.
- Bake the tart for 25-30 minutes, or until the crust is firm and the filling is bubbly.
- Let the tart cool before slicing and serving.

<u>VEGAN GRANOLA CUPS</u>

Ingredients:

- 2 cups rolled oats
- 1 cup shredded coconut
- 1/2 cup chopped almonds
- 1/4 cup maple syrup
- 1/4 cup coconut oil
- 1 tsp vanilla extract
- 1/4 tsp salt

Directions:

- Preheat your oven to 350°F (175°C).
- In a large mixing bowl, combine the oats, shredded coconut, and chopped almonds. Mix well.
- In a separate mixing bowl, combine the maple syrup, coconut oil, vanilla extract, and salt. Mix well.
- Pour the wet ingredients into the dry ingredients and mix until the oats are evenly coated.
- Grease a 12-cup muffin tin with non-stick spray.
- Using a spoon or cookie scoop, press the granola mixture into the cups of the muffin tin. Press it firmly and evenly.
- Bake the granola cups for 10-15 minutes, or until they are golden brown.
- Remove the granola cups from the oven and let them cool before removing them from the muffin tin.

- Note: Feel free to mix and match ingredients to your taste, adding or removing ingredients as you like.

<u>DAIRY-FREE AND GLUTEN-FREE CARROT CAKE</u>

Ingredients:

- 1 cup almond flour
- 1 cup gluten-free oat flour
- 1 tsp baking powder
- 1 tsp baking soda
- 1 tsp cinnamon
- 1/2 tsp nutmeg
- 1/2 tsp ginger
- 1/2 tsp salt
- 3/4 cup coconut sugar
- 3/4 cup unsweetened applesauce
- 1/2 cup dairy-free milk
- 1/4 cup coconut oil, melted
- 2 tsp vanilla extract
- 2 cups grated carrots
- 1/2 cup chopped pecans (optional)

Directions:

- Preheat the oven to 350°F (175°C). Grease a 9-inch round cake pan or line it with parchment paper.
- In a large mixing bowl, combine the almond flour, oat flour, baking powder, baking soda, cinnamon, nutmeg, ginger, and salt. Mix well.
- In a separate mixing bowl, combine the coconut sugar, applesauce, dairy-free milk, coconut oil, and vanilla extract. Mix well.

- Gradually add the wet ingredients to the dry ingredients and mix until just combined.
- Fold in the grated carrots and chopped pecans (if using).
- Into the prepared cake pan, pour the batter.
- Bake the cake for 35-40 minutes or until a toothpick inserted into the center comes out clean.
- Let the cake cool in the pan for 10-15 minutes before removing it from the pan and letting it cool completely on a wire rack.
- You can also frost it with a dairy-free cream cheese frosting or a dairy-free buttercream frosting.

Note: If you are not gluten-intolerant, you can use wheat flour instead of gluten-free oat flour.

<u>DAIRY-FREE BANANA CHOCOLATE ICE CREAM</u>

Ingredients:

- 4 ripe bananas
- 1/2 cup dairy-free chocolate chips
- 1 tsp vanilla extract

Directions:

- Peel and slice the bananas, then place them in a ziplock bag or container and freeze for at least 2 hours.
- Once the bananas are frozen, place them in a food processor or high-speed blender.
- Blend the frozen bananas until they become creamy and smooth. It may take a few minutes and you may need to stop and scrape down the sides of the bowl a few times.
- Once the banana is creamy and smooth, add the dairy-free chocolate chips and vanilla extract. Blend until the chocolate is fully incorporated.
- Transfer the ice cream to a container and freeze for at least 2 hours, or until it is firm.
- Scoop the ice cream into bowls and enjoy!

GLUTEN-FREE AND DAIRY-FREE BLUEBERRY CUPCAKES

Ingredients:

- 1 1/2 cups gluten-free flour blend
- 1 tsp baking powder
- 1/2 tsp baking soda
- 1/4 tsp salt
- 1/2 cup coconut sugar
- 1/2 cup unsweetened applesauce
- 1/4 cup dairy-free milk
- 1/4 cup coconut oil, melted
- 2 tsp vanilla extract
- 1 cup fresh blueberries

Directions:

- Preheat your oven to 350°F (175°C).
- With paper liners, line a 12-cup muffin tin.
- In a large mixing bowl, combine the gluten-free flour blend, baking powder, baking soda, and salt. Mix well.
- In a separate mixing bowl, combine the coconut sugar, applesauce, dairy-free milk, coconut oil, and vanilla extract. Mix well.
- Gradually add the wet ingredients to the dry ingredients and mix until just combined.
- Fold in the blueberries gently.
- Divide the batter evenly among the cups of the muffin tin.

- Bake the cupcakes for 20-25 minutes or until a toothpick inserted into the center comes out clean.
- Let the cupcakes cool in the pan for 10-15 minutes before removing them from the pan and letting them cool completely on a wire rack.

You can also frost them with a dairy-free cream cheese frosting or a dairy-free buttercream frosting.

VEGAN AND GLUTEN-FREE CHOCOLATE HAZELNUT SPREAD

Ingredients:

- 1 cup hazelnuts
- 1/2 cup cacao powder
- 1/4 cup maple syrup
- 1/4 cup coconut oil, melted
- 1 tsp vanilla extract
- Pinch of salt

Directions:

- Preheat the oven to 350°F (175°C). Spread the hazelnuts on a baking sheet and roast for 10-15 minutes, or until the skins start to crack.
- Remove the hazelnuts from the oven and wrap in a clean kitchen towel. Rub the hazelnuts together to remove as much of the skin as possible.
- Once the hazelnuts are cool, place them in a food processor and blend until they become a smooth paste.
- Add the cacao powder, maple syrup, coconut oil, vanilla extract, and salt to the hazelnut paste. Blend until smooth.
- Transfer the spread to an airtight container and store in the refrigerator for up to 1 month.

VEGAN AND GLUTEN-FREE TOFU CHOCOLATE CAKES

Ingredients:

- 1 block of firm tofu
- 1/2 cup gluten-free flour
- 1/2 cup cacao powder
- 1/2 cup maple syrup
- 1/4 cup vegetable oil
- 2 tsp vanilla extract
- 1 tsp baking powder
- Pinch of salt

Directions:

- Preheat the oven to 350°F (175°C). Grease a 6-cup muffin tin with non-stick spray.
- Drain the tofu properly and press it between two paper towels to remove any excess water.
- Place the tofu in a food processor and blend until it becomes a smooth puree.
- In a large mixing bowl, combine the flour, cacao powder, baking powder, and salt. Mix well.
- In a separate mixing bowl, combine the maple syrup, vegetable oil, and vanilla extract. Mix well.
- Gradually add the wet ingredients to the dry ingredients and mix until just combined.
- Fold in the tofu puree until well combined.
- Divide the batter evenly among the cups of the muffin tin.

- Bake the cakes for 20-25 minutes or until a toothpick inserted into the center comes out clean.
- Let the cakes cool in the pan for 10-15 minutes before removing them from the pan and letting them cool completely on a wire rack.

VEGAN AND GLUTEN-FREE PINK LEMONADE CUPCAKES

Ingredients:

- 1 1/2 cups gluten-free flour blend
- 1 tsp baking powder
- 1/2 tsp baking soda
- 1/4 tsp salt
- 1/2 cup coconut sugar
- 1/2 cup unsweetened applesauce
- 1/4 cup almond milk
- 1/4 cup coconut oil, melted
- 2 tsp vanilla extract
- 2 tsp pink lemonade powder
- Pink food coloring (optional)

Directions:

- Preheat the oven to 350°F (175°C). Line a 12-cup muffin tin with paper liners.
- In a large mixing bowl, combine the gluten-free flour blend, baking powder, baking soda, and salt. Mix well.
- In a separate mixing bowl, combine the coconut sugar, applesauce, almond milk, coconut oil, vanilla extract, pink lemonade powder, and food coloring (if using). Mix well.
- Gradually add the wet ingredients to the dry ingredients and mix until just combined.

- Divide the batter evenly among the cups of the muffin tin.
- Bake the cupcakes for 20-25 minutes or until a toothpick inserted into the center comes out clean.
- Let the cupcakes cool in the pan for 10-15 minutes before removing them from the pan and letting them cool completely on a wire rack.
- Serve the cupcakes as it is or you can frost them with a dairy-free cream cheese frosting or a dairy-free buttercream frosting.

Note: The pink lemonade powder can be found in most grocery stores and online. If you cannot find it, you can use lemon zest and juice for the lemon flavor.

AUTUMNAL VEGAN CARROTS WITH WALNUTS

Ingredients:

- 2 lbs carrots, peeled and sliced
- 1/2 cup walnuts, chopped
- 2 tbsp olive oil
- 2 tbsp maple syrup
- 1 tsp ground cinnamon
- 1/2 tsp ground ginger
- 1/4 tsp ground nutmeg
- Salt and pepper, to taste

Directions:

- Preheat your oven to 400°F (200°C).
- In a large mixing bowl, combine the carrots, walnuts, olive oil, maple syrup, cinnamon, ginger, nutmeg, salt, and pepper. Toss the mixture until the carrots are evenly coated.
- Spread the carrot mixture on a baking sheet in a single layer.
- Roast the carrots for 25-30 minutes, or until they are tender and lightly browned.
- Serve the roasted carrots as a side dish or top them with additional chopped walnuts for garnish.

<u>JAVA BANANAS</u>

Ingredients:

- 2 ripe bananas
- 1/2 cup strong coffee
- 1 tbsp maple syrup
- 1 tsp vanilla extract

Directions:

- Peel and slice the bananas.
- In a small mixing bowl, combine the coffee, maple syrup, and vanilla extract. Mix well.
- In a separate pan or skillet, bring the coffee mixture to a simmer over medium heat.
- Add the banana slices to the pan and cook them for 2-3 minutes per side, or until they are heated through.
- Serve the java bananas over ice cream or yogurt, or topped with whipped cream.

SWEET DESSERT BLISS

Ingredients:

- 1 can full-fat coconut milk
- 1/4 cup maple syrup
- 1 tsp vanilla extract
- 1/4 tsp salt
- 2 cups fresh berries (strawberries, raspberries, blueberries, etc.)

Directions:

- In a medium saucepan, combine the coconut milk, maple syrup, vanilla extract, and salt.
- Heat the mixture over medium heat until it begins to simmer.
- Remove the pan from the heat and let it cool for a few minutes.
- Pour the mixture into a blender and blend until smooth and creamy.
- Divide the mixture into individual bowls and top with fresh berries.
- Serve the dessert chilled.

Note: You can also add other ingredients such as chocolate chips, nuts, and different types of fruits to make it more appealing.

<u>GLUTEN-FREE AND DAIRY-FREE APPLE CRUMB</u>

Ingredients:

- 4 cups of peeled and diced apples
- 1/2 cup gluten-free flour blend
- 1/2 cup rolled oats
- 1/2 cup brown sugar
- 1/4 cup coconut oil, melted
- 1 tsp cinnamon
- 1 tsp vanilla extract
- Pinch of salt

Directions:

- Preheat the oven to 350°F (175°C). Grease a 9-inch square baking dish with non-stick spray.
- In a large mixing bowl, combine the apples, cinnamon, and vanilla extract. Mix well.
- Transfer the apple mixture to the prepared baking dish.
- In a separate mixing bowl, combine the flour blend, rolled oats, brown sugar, coconut oil, and salt. Mix well.
- Sprinkle the crumb mixture over the apples.
- Bake the apple crumb for 30-35 minutes or until the apples are tender and the crumb is golden brown.
- Serve the apple crumb warm or at room temperature.

<u>DAIRY-FREE CUSTARD</u>

Ingredients:

- 2 cups almond milk
- 1/2 cup sugar
- 3 tbsp cornstarch
- 1/4 tsp salt
- 2 tsp vanilla extract

Directions:

- In a medium saucepan, combine the almond milk, sugar, cornstarch, and salt. Whisk until the mixture is smooth.
- Heat the mixture over medium heat, whisking constantly, until it thickens and comes to a simmer.
- Remove the pan from the heat and stir in the vanilla extract.
- Let the custard cool for a few minutes before pouring it into a bowl or individual cups.
- Cover the custard with plastic wrap, pressing the wrap directly onto the surface of the custard to prevent a skin from forming.
- Chill the custard in the refrigerator for at least 2 hours, or until it is cold and set.

FRIED HONEY BANANAS

Ingredients:

- 4 ripe bananas
- 1/4 cup coconut oil
- 1/4 cup honey
- 1 tsp vanilla extract
- Pinch of salt

Directions:

- Peel and slice the bananas.
- In a large skillet or pan, heat the coconut oil over medium heat.
- Combine the honey, vanilla extract, and salt in a small mixing bowl. Mix well.
- Add the banana slices to the skillet and cook them for 2-3 minutes per side, or until they are golden brown.
- Remove the bananas and drain them on a paper towel-lined plate.
- Drizzle the honey mixture over the bananas.
- Serve the fried honey bananas warm or at room temperature.

Note: You can also add additional toppings such as chopped nuts, coconut flakes, or chocolate chips for extra flavor and texture. If you prefer a sweeter dish you can add more honey or any sweetener of your preference.

<u>AVOCADO SORBET</u>

Ingredients:

- 2 ripe avocados
- 1 cup sugar
- 1 cup water
- 1/4 cup lime juice

Directions:

- In a medium-sized saucepan, combine the water and sugar and bring to a boil over medium heat. Stir until the sugar has dissolved, then remove from heat and let cool.
- Peel the avocados and remove the pit, then puree them in a blender or food processor.
- Stir in the cooled sugar syrup and lime juice, then transfer the mixture to an ice cream maker and churn according to the manufacturer's directions.
- Freeze the sorbet for at least 2 hours before serving, or until firm.

BANANA CUPCAKES

Ingredients:

- 1 1/2 cups all-purpose flour
- 1 tsp baking powder
- 1/2 tsp baking soda
- 1/4 tsp salt
- 1/2 cup unsalted butter, at room temperature
- 1 cup sugar
- 2 eggs
- 1 tsp vanilla extract
- 1 cup mashed ripe banana (about 2 medium)

Directions:

- Preheat the oven to 350°F (180°C) and line a 12-cup muffin tin with paper liners.
- In a medium bowl, whisk together the baking powder, flour, salt and baking soda.
- In a large bowl, beat the butter and sugar together until light and fluffy. Beat in the eggs one by one, and then stir in the vanilla and mashed banana.
- Gradually add the flour mixture to the banana mixture, stirring just until combined.
- Divide the batter among the muffin cups and bake for 18-20 minutes, or until a toothpick inserted into the center of a cupcake comes out clean.
- Let the cupcakes cool in the pan for 5 minutes, then transfer them to a wire rack to cool completely.

<u>FLOURLESS CHOCOLATE CAKE</u>

Ingredients:

- 1 cup (2 sticks) unsalted butter
- 1/4 cup unsweetened cocoa powder
- 1 1/4 cups granulated sugar
- 1/4 teaspoon salt
- 1 cup semi-sweet chocolate chips
- 1 teaspoon of vanilla extract
- 4 large eggs

Directions:

- Preheat the oven to 350°F (180°C). Grease a 9-inch round cake pan with butter and dust with cocoa powder.
- Melt the butter over medium heat in a medium saucepan. Remove from heat and stir in the sugar, cocoa powder, salt, and vanilla extract.
- Add the eggs, one at a time, stirring well after each addition. Stir in the chocolate chips.
- Pour the batter into the pan prepared earlier and bake for about 25-30 minutes.
- Insert a toothpick into the center, pull it out and observe occasionally. The cake is ready when the toothpick inserted into the center comes out clean.
- Let the cake first cool in the pan for 10 minutes, then turn it out onto a wire rack to cool completely.

<u>EGGLESS HONEY CAKE</u>

Ingredients:

- 2 cups all-purpose flour
- 2 tsp baking powder
- 1/2 tsp baking soda
- 1/2 tsp cinnamon powder
- 1/4 tsp nutmeg powder
- 1/4 tsp allspice powder
- 1/4 tsp ground ginger
- 1/2 cup honey
- 1/2 cup vegetable oil
- 1/2 cup milk
- 1 tsp vanilla extract

Directions:

- Preheat your oven to 350°F (180°C). Grease and flour a 9x5 inch loaf pan.
- In a medium bowl, whisk together the baking powder, flour, cinnamon powder, baking soda, allspice powder, nutmeg powder, and ginger.
- In a separate bowl, mix together the honey, oil, milk, and vanilla extract.
- Add the dry ingredients to the wet ingredients gradually and mix until it is evenly combined.
- Pour the batter into the already prepared pan and bake for about 40-45 minutes.

- Insert a toothpick into the center, pull it out and observe occasionally. The cake is ready when the toothpick inserted into the center comes out clean.
- Let the cake first cool in the pan for 10 minutes, then turn it out onto a wire rack to cool completely.

<u>CHRISTMAS IN A CUP</u>

Ingredients:

- 2 cups boiling water
- 1 cup dried cranberries
- 1/2 cup currants
- 1/2 cup dried, chopped apricots
- 1/2 cup dried apples, chopped
- 1/2 cup raisins
- 1/2 cup honey
- 1 cinnamon stick
- 1 tsp vanilla extract
- 1 cup all-purpose flour
- 1 tsp baking powder
- 1/4 tsp baking soda
- 1/4 tsp salt
- 1/4 cup unsalted butter, at room temperature
- 1/2 cup granulated sugar
- 1 egg

Directions:

- In a large bowl, combine the boiling water, cranberries, apricots, apples, raisins, currants, honey, cinnamon stick, and vanilla extract. Let stand for 30 minutes to allow the fruits to soften.
- Preheat the oven to 350°F (180°C) and line a 12-cup muffin tin with paper liners.
- In a medium bowl, whisk together the flour, baking powder, baking soda, and salt.

- In a large bowl, beat the butter and sugar together until light and fluffy. Beat in the egg, then stir in the fruit mixture.
- Gradually add the flour mixture to the fruit mixture, stirring just until combined.
- Divide the batter among the muffin cups and bake for 18-20 minutes, or until a toothpick inserted into the center of a cupcake comes out clean.
- Let the cupcakes cool in the pan for 5 minutes, then transfer them to a wire rack to cool completely.

<u>BROWNIE BITES</u>

Ingredients:

- 1/2 cup all-purpose flour
- 1/2 cup unsweetened cocoa powder
- 1/4 tsp baking powder
- 1/4 tsp salt
- 1/2 cup semi-sweet chocolate chips
- 1/2 cup unsalted butter, melted
- 1 cup granulated sugar
- 1 tsp vanilla extract
- 2 eggs

Directions:

- Preheat the oven to 350°F (180°C) and line a mini muffin tin with paper liners.
- In a medium bowl, whisk together the cocoa powder, flour, salt and baking powder.
- In a large bowl, mix together the melted butter, sugar, vanilla extract and eggs.
- Gradually add the dry ingredients to the wet ingredients and mix until well combined. Stir in the chocolate chips.
- Using a small cookie scoop or spoon, fill each muffin cup about 2/3 full with batter.
- Bake for 12-15 minutes, or until a toothpick inserted into the center of a brownie bite comes out clean.
- Let the brownie bites cool in the pan for 5 minutes, then transfer them to a wire rack to cool completely.

- Enjoy your delicious homemade Brownie Bites!

<u>BLUEBERRY GALETTE</u>

Ingredients:

- 1 1/4 cups all-purpose flour
- 1/4 tsp salt
- 1/2 cup (1 stick) cold unsalted butter, cut into small pieces
- 2-3 tbsp ice water
- 2 cups fresh blueberries
- 1/4 cup granulated sugar
- 1 tbsp cornstarch
- 1 tbsp fresh lemon juice
- 1 egg beaten with 1 tsp water, for egg wash
- coarse sugar, for sprinkling

Directions:

- In a large bowl, whisk together the salt and flour. Using a pastry cutter or your fingers, cut in the butter until the mixture resembles coarse crumbs.
- Gradually add the ice water, 1 tablespoon at a time, until the dough comes together. Gather the dough into a ball, flatten it into a disk, and wrap it in plastic wrap. Chill for at least 1 hour.
- Preheat your oven to 425°F (220°C). Roll out the dough on a lightly floured surface into a 12-inch round.
- In a medium bowl, toss together the blueberries, sugar, cornstarch, and lemon juice.

- Arrange the blueberry mixture in the center of the dough round, leaving a 2-inch border. Fold the border up and over the filling, pleating the edge to make it fit.
- Brush the crust with the egg wash and sprinkle with coarse sugar.
- Place the galette on a baking sheet and bake for 25-30 minutes, or until the crust is golden brown and the filling is bubbly. Let cool before serving.

ROYAL CROWN PIE

Ingredients:

- 1 pie crust
- 1/2 cup granulated sugar
- 1/4 cup cornstarch
- 1/4 tsp salt
- 3 cups of mixed berries (raspberries, blueberries, blackberries, etc)
- 1 egg white, beaten
- 1/4 cup coarse sugar

Directions:

- Preheat your oven to 375°F (190°C). Roll out the pie crust and press it into a 9-inch pie dish. Trim the edges and set aside.
- In a medium-sized saucepan, whisk together the cornstarch, sugar, and salt. Add the mixed berries and stir to coat. Cook the mixture over medium heat, stirring frequently, until it comes to a boil. Cook for an additional 2 minutes, or until thickened.
- Pour the berry mixture into the prepared crust and spread it out evenly.
- Cut the remaining pie dough into 1/2-inch wide strips. Arrange the strips in a lattice pattern on top of the filling.
- Brush the crust with the beaten egg white and sprinkle with coarse sugar.

- Bake the pie for 45-50 minutes, or until the crust is golden brown and the filling is bubbly. Let cool before serving.

MOCHA RICOTTA CRÉME

Ingredients:

- 1 cup part-skim ricotta cheese
- 1/4 cup granulated sugar
- 1 tsp unsweetened cocoa powder
- 1 tsp instant coffee granules
- 1 tsp vanilla extract
- 1/4 tsp salt

Directions:

- In a medium bowl, combine the ricotta cheese, sugar, instant coffee granules, cocoa powder, vanilla extract, and salt.
- Using an electric mixer, beat the mixture on medium-high speed until smooth and creamy, about 2-3 minutes.
- Taste and adjust sweetness or coffee flavor as needed.
- Cover and refrigerate the crème for at least 1 hour, or until chilled and firm.
- Serve the mocha ricotta crème as a dessert or use as a filling for cakes, tarts, or pastries.
- Enjoy your delicious homemade Mocha Ricotta Crème!

ORANGE MUFFINS

Ingredients:

- 2 cups all-purpose flour
- 1/2 cup granulated sugar
- 2 tsp baking powder
- 1/2 tsp salt
- 1/2 cup unsalted butter, melted
- 2 eggs
- 1/2 cup milk
- 1/2 cup fresh orange juice
- 1 tsp orange zest

Directions:

- Preheat the oven to 400°F (200°C) and line a 12-cup muffin tin with paper liners.
- In a large bowl, whisk together the flour, baking powder, salt and sugar.
- In a separate bowl, mix together the melted butter, eggs, milk, orange juice, and orange zest.
- Gradually add the wet ingredients to the dry ingredients and mix until just combined.
- Divide the batter among the muffin cups and bake for 18-20 minutes, or until a toothpick inserted into the center of a muffin comes out clean.
- First allow the muffins to cool in the pan for 5 minutes, then transfer them to a wire rack to cool completely.

- Enjoy your homemade orange muffins, they are delicious and perfect for breakfast or brunch.

CHAPTER SEVEN

Snacks

<u>COOKIE CUP TARTS</u>

Ingredients:

- 1 cup all-purpose flour
- 1/2 cup unsalted butter, at room temperature
- 1/4 cup granulated sugar
- 1/4 tsp salt
- 1/2 tsp vanilla extract
- 1 egg yolk
- 1/2 cup your favorite jam or preserves

Directions:

- Preheat the oven to 350°F (180°C) and line a 12-cup muffin tin with paper liners.
- In a medium bowl, whisk together the flour, butter, sugar, salt, vanilla extract, and egg yolk until a dough forms.
- Using a small cookie scoop or spoon, press a heaping tablespoon of dough into the bottom and up the sides of each muffin cup.
- Fill each dough-lined cup with a tablespoon of your favorite jam or preserves.
- Bake the tarts for 15-20 minutes, or until the edges are golden brown. Let cool in the pan for 5 minutes before removing to a wire rack to cool completely.

FRUIT AND GINGER POPSICLES

Ingredients:

- 1 cup mixed berries (strawberries, raspberries, blueberries, etc)
- 1/2 cup pineapple chunks
- 1/2 cup orange juice
- 1/4 cup honey
- 2 tbsp grated fresh ginger

Directions:

- In a blender, combine the mixed berries, pineapple, orange juice, honey, and grated ginger. Blend until smooth.
- Pour the mixture into Popsicle molds and freeze until it is firm for about 4-6 hours.
- To remove the popsicles from the molds, run them under warm water for a few seconds before gently pulling them out.

<u>YOGURT BITES</u>

Ingredients:

- 2 cups plain Greek yogurt
- 1/4 cup honey
- 1 tsp vanilla extract
- 1/2 cup fresh berries or chopped fruit

Directions:

- In a medium bowl, mix together the yogurt, honey, and vanilla extract until well combined.
- Fold in the fresh berries or chopped fruit.
- Using a small cookie scoop or spoon, drop the mixture onto a parchment-lined baking sheet or silicone mat.
- Freeze for about 2 hours, or until firm.
- Store the yogurt bites in an airtight container in the freezer for up to 2 weeks.

<u>BAKED MUSHROOM SNACKS</u>

Ingredients:

- 1 pound cremini mushrooms, cleaned and stemmed
- 2 cloves garlic, minced
- 2 tbsp olive oil
- 1/4 cup of grated Parmesan cheese
- Salt and pepper, to taste

Directions:

- Preheat your oven to 400°F (200°C).
- In a large bowl, toss the mushrooms with garlic, olive oil, salt, and pepper.
- Arrange the mushrooms on a baking sheet and bake for 20-25 minutes, or until they are tender and golden brown.
- Remove the mushrooms from the oven and sprinkle them with Parmesan cheese.
- Return the mushrooms to the oven and bake for an additional 5 minutes, or until the cheese is melted and bubbly.
- Serve the mushrooms as a snack, or as a side dish with your favorite protein.

<u>CHILI CHICKPEAS</u>

Ingredients:

- 1 (15 oz) can chickpeas, drained and rinsed
- 1 tbsp olive oil
- 1 tsp chili powder
- 1/2 tsp ground cumin
- 1/4 tsp garlic powder
- Salt and pepper, to taste

Directions:

- Preheat the oven to 400°F (200°C).
- In a large bowl, toss the chickpeas with olive oil, chili powder, cumin, garlic powder, salt, and pepper.
- Spread the chickpeas out in a single layer on a baking sheet.
- Bake for 20-25 minutes, or until crispy and golden brown.
- Serve the chili chickpeas as a snack, or as a topping for salads or grain bowls.

<u>PEANUT BUTTER SNACK</u>

Ingredients:

- 1 cup rolled oats
- 1/2 cup peanut butter
- 1/4 cup honey
- 1/4 cup chopped peanuts

Directions:

- In a medium bowl, mix together the oats, peanut butter, and honey until well combined.
- Stir in the chopped peanuts.
- Roll the mixture into balls, about 1 tablespoon each.
- Refrigerate the balls for at least 1 hour, or until firm.

<u>PITA SNACKS</u>

Ingredients:

- 1/4 cup olive oil
- 2 cloves garlic, minced
- 1 tsp dried oregano
- 1/2 tsp red pepper flakes (optional)
- Salt and pepper, to taste
- 4 pita breads

Directions:

- Preheat your oven to 350°F (175°C).
- In a small bowl, mix together olive oil, garlic, oregano, red pepper flakes (if using), salt, and pepper.
- Brush the mixture evenly over the pita breads.
- Cut the pita breads into wedges and place them on a baking sheet.
- Bake for 10-12 minutes, or until golden brown and crispy.
- Serve with hummus or your favorite dip.

CHEESY POTATO FRITTATA

Ingredients:

- 1 tbsp olive oil
- 1 onion, diced
- 2 cloves garlic, minced
- 3 cups diced potatoes
- 1/4 tsp salt
- 1/4 tsp black pepper
- 1/4 tsp paprika
- 1/4 cup chopped fresh parsley
- 8 eggs
- 1/2 cup grated cheddar cheese

Directions:

- First, heat the olive oil in a skillet over medium heat. Add the onion and garlic and sauté for 2-3 minutes, or until softened.
- Add the diced potatoes, salt, pepper, and paprika, and cook for 10-15 minutes, or until the potatoes are cooked through and tender.
- Whisk together the eggs and parsley in a bowl.
- Pour the egg mixture over the potato mixture in the skillet and cook for 2-3 minutes, or until the edges begin to set.
- Sprinkle the grated cheese over the top of the frittata and transfer the skillet to the oven.
- Broil for 2-3 minutes, or until the cheese is melted and the eggs are set.

- Let the frittata cool for a few minutes before slicing and serving.

<u>HAYSTACK YUMMY</u>

Ingredients:

- 1 bag of butterscotch chips
- 1 bag of chocolate chips
- 1 bag of chow mein noodles

Directions:

- In a microwave-safe bowl, melt the butterscotch chips and chocolate chips in 30-second increments, stirring in between, until smooth.
- Stir in chow mein noodles until evenly coated.
- Drop spoonfuls of the mixture onto a parchment-lined baking sheet.
- Allow the haystacks to set up in the refrigerator for about 30 minutes.

<u>CRISPY RICE SNACKS</u>

Ingredients:

- 4 cups crispy rice cereal
- 1/4 cup butter
- 1/4 cup honey
- 1 tsp vanilla extract
- 1/4 tsp salt

Directions:

- In a large saucepan, melt the butter over medium heat. Stir in the honey, vanilla extract, and salt.
- Remove the pan from the heat and add the crispy rice cereal, stirring until well coated.
- Spread the mixture out onto a baking sheet lined with parchment paper.
- Press down on the mixture to compact it slightly.
- Let it cool completely, and then break it into bite-size pieces.

<u>GLUTEN-FREE TRAIL MIX</u>

Ingredients:

- 1 cup gluten-free rolled oats
- 1/2 cup pumpkin seeds
- 1/2 cup sunflower seeds
- 1/2 cup dried cranberries
- 1/2 cup raisins
- 1/2 cup chopped almonds
- 1/4 cup unsweetened shredded coconut
- 1/4 cup dark chocolate chips

Directions:

- In a large bowl, combine the oats, pumpkin seeds, sunflower seeds, dried cranberries, raisins, chopped almonds, shredded coconut, and chocolate chips.
- Mix well to combine.
- Store the trail mix in an airtight container at room temperature for up to 1 month.

<u>COCONUT BALLS</u>

Ingredients:

- 1 cup shredded coconut
- 1/2 cup sweetened condensed milk
- 1 tsp vanilla extract

Directions:

- In a medium bowl, mix together the shredded coconut, sweetened condensed milk, and vanilla extract until well combined.
- Roll the mixture into small balls, about 1 inch in diameter.
- Place the balls on a baking sheet lined with parchment paper and refrigerate for at least 30 minutes to firm up.
- Store the coconut balls in an airtight container in the refrigerator for up to a week.

BUFFALO CHICKEN DIP

Ingredients:

- 2 cups shredded cooked chicken
- 1 cup buffalo wing sauce
- 8 oz cream cheese, softened
- 1/2 cup of shredded cheddar cheese
- 1/2 cup sour cream
- 1/2 cup ranch dressing
- Optional toppings: blue cheese crumbles, chopped green onions

Directions:

- Preheat the oven to 350 degrees F.
- In a large bowl, combine the buffalo wing sauce, shredded chicken, cream cheese, ranch dressing, sour cream, and cheddar cheese. Stir until it is evenly combined.
- Transfer the mixture to a baking dish and spread it out evenly.
- Bake the dip for 20-25 minutes, or until it's hot and bubbly.
- Serve the dip with your choice of toppings, and enjoy with tortilla chips, crackers, or veggies.

CHOCOLATE CHIA BALLS

Ingredients:

- 1/2 cup chia seeds
- 1/2 cup almond butter
- 1/4 cup unsweetened cocoa powder
- 1/4 cup honey
- 1 tsp vanilla extract
- 1/4 cup chocolate chips
- pinch of salt

Directions:

- In a large mixing bowl, stir together the chia seeds, almond butter, cocoa powder, honey, vanilla extract, chocolate chips and salt.
- Mix until well combined and a dough-like consistency is formed.
- Using a cookie scoop or spoon, form dough into small balls.
- Place on a baking sheet and chill in the fridge for 30 minutes.
- Store in an airtight container in the refrigerator for up to 1 week.

<u>SWEET POTATO HUMMUS</u>

Ingredients:

- 1 medium-sized sweet potato, peeled and chopped
- 1 can (15 oz) chickpeas, drained and rinsed
- 2 cloves garlic
- 2 tbsp tahini
- 2 tbsp lemon juice
- 1 tsp ground cumin
- Salt and pepper, to taste
- Olive oil, for drizzling

Directions:

- Preheat the oven to 400°F. Place the sweet potato on a baking sheet and drizzle with a little bit of olive oil. Roast for 20-25 minutes, or until tender.
- In a food processor, combine the sweet potato, chickpeas, garlic, tahini, lemon juice, cumin, salt, and pepper. Process until smooth.
- Taste and adjust the seasonings as required. Serve with veggies or pita chips.

<u>ZUCCHINI CHIPS</u>

Ingredients:

- 2 medium zucchinis, thinly sliced
- 1/4 cup all-purpose flour
- 1/4 cup grated Parmesan cheese
- 1/4 tsp garlic powder
- Salt and pepper, to taste
- Olive oil, for drizzling

Directions:

- Preheat the oven to 425°F, and line a baking sheet with parchment paper.
- In a shallow dish, combine the flour, Parmesan cheese, garlic powder, salt and pepper.
- Dip each zucchini slice in the flour mixture, pressing to coat both sides. Place on the baking sheet that you prepared earlier.
- Drizzle with a little bit of olive oil.
- Bake for 15-20 minutes, or until golden brown and crispy.

<u>CARAMEL ENERGY BITES</u>

Ingredients:

- 1 cup rolled oats
- 1/2 cup almond butter
- 1/4 cup honey
- 2 tbsp ground flaxseed
- 2 tbsp chia seeds
- 1 tsp vanilla extract
- 1/2 tsp salt
- 1/2 cup caramel bits

Directions:

- In a medium bowl, combine the oats, almond butter, honey, flaxseed, chia seeds, vanilla extract and salt. Mix until well combined.
- Stir in the caramel bits.
- Roll the mixture into balls, about 1 inch in diameter.
- Refrigerate for at least 30 minutes, or until firm.
- Enjoy your snacks!

<u>COCONUT TOFU TENDERS</u>

Ingredients:

- 14 oz extra-firm tofu, pressed and cut into 1/2-inch slices
- 1/2 cup flour
- 1/2 tsp salt
- 1/4 tsp black pepper
- 1/2 cup unsweetened shredded coconut
- 1/2 cup panko breadcrumbs
- 1/4 cup of vegetable oil

Directions:

- Combine the flour, pepper and salt in a shallow dish.
- In another shallow dish, combine the shredded coconut and breadcrumbs.
- Dip each tofu slice first into the flour mixture, then into the coconut mixture, pressing the coconut mixture onto the tofu to adhere.
- Heat the vegetable oil over medium-high heat in a large skillet.
- Add the coated tofu slices to the skillet and fry for 2-3 minutes on each side, until golden brown.
- Drain on a paper towel-lined plate and serve warm.

<u>FALAFEL</u>

Ingredients:

- 1 cup dried chickpeas, soaked overnight
- 1/2 cup parsley, chopped
- 1/2 cup cilantro, chopped
- 1 onion, chopped
- 3 cloves garlic, minced
- 1 tsp cumin
- 1 tsp coriander
- 1/2 tsp salt
- 1/4 tsp black pepper
- 1/4 cup flour
- Vegetable oil, for frying

Directions:

- Drain and rinse the soaked chickpeas, then add them to a food processor along with the parsley, cilantro, onion, garlic, cumin, coriander, salt, and pepper.
- Pulse until the mixture is well combined but still slightly chunky.
- Add the flour and pulse again until the mixture forms a thick paste.
- Form the mixture into small, flattened balls (about 1 1/2 inches in diameter).
- Heat the oil over medium-high heat in a large skillet.

- Add the falafel balls to the skillet and fry for 2-3 minutes on each side, until golden brown.
- Drain on a paper towel-lined plate and serve warm with tahini sauce or yogurt sauce.

<u>SWEDE (RUTABAGA) CHIPS</u>

Ingredients:

- 1 large swede, peeled and thinly sliced
- 2 tablespoon olive oil
- Salt and pepper to taste

Directions:

- Preheat the oven to 400F.
- Toss the swede slices in olive oil and season with salt and pepper.
- Spread the swede slices out in a single layer on a baking sheet.
- Bake for 15-20 minutes, flipping the slices halfway through, until they are golden brown and crispy.
- Remove from the oven and let cool for a few minutes before serving.

<u>SPICY PINEAPPLE SALSA</u>

Ingredients:

- 1 pineapple, peeled and diced
- 1 jalapeño, seeded and diced
- 1/2 red onion, diced
- 1/4 cup cilantro, chopped
- 1 lime, juiced
- Salt and pepper, to taste

Directions:

- In a large bowl, combine the pineapple, jalapeño, red onion, and cilantro.
- Stir in the lime juice and season with salt and pepper to taste.
- Refrigerate for at least 30 minutes to allow the flavors to meld before serving.
- Serve with tortilla chips or as a topping for grilled chicken or fish.

Note: The recipe for the Spicy Pineapple Salsa contains jalapeño, which is a type of chili pepper that can be spicy for some people, and may cause discomfort for those with Ulcerative colitis. However, you can adjust the recipe to your liking by using less jalapeño or not using it at all.

It's always a good idea to check with your doctor or a registered dietitian to see what specific foods and dietary restrictions are best for you. They may also provide a list of

foods that you should avoid or limit and give you advice on
how to manage your condition through diet and nutrition.

ANGEL HAIR PASTA WITH LEMON AND PARMESAN

Ingredients:

- 8 oz angel hair pasta
- 2 cloves garlic, minced
- 1/4 cup grated Parmesan cheese
- 2 tbsp olive oil
- 1/4 tsp salt
- 1/4 tsp black pepper
- 2 tbsp lemon juice
- 2 tbsp chopped parsley

Directions:

- Cook the pasta according to the package instructions.
- Drain and set aside.
- In a pan, heat the olive oil over medium heat.
- Add the sauté and garlic until fragrant.
- Add the cooked pasta and toss to coat in the oil and garlic.
- Add the Parmesan cheese, salt, pepper, and lemon juice and toss again.
- Serve the pasta in bowls, and garnish with parsley.

<u>NICE CREAM SUNDAE</u>

Ingredients:

- 2 frozen ripe bananas, peeled and diced
- 1/4 cup Nut milk
- 2 tbsp honey or maple syrup
- 1 tsp vanilla extract
- Toppings of your choice (e.g., chocolate chips, nuts, berries, coconut flakes)

Directions:

- In a food processor or blender, combine the frozen bananas, milk, honey or maple syrup, and vanilla extract.
- Blend until smooth and creamy, scraping down the sides as needed.
- Scoop the nice cream into bowls or cones and add toppings of your choice.
- Serve immediately and enjoy!

<u>GARDEN FRITTATA</u>

Ingredients:

- 6 eggs
- 1/4 cup milk
- Salt and pepper, to taste
- tbsp olive oil
- 1/2 onion, diced
- 1/4 cup of grated Parmesan cheese
- 1 red bell pepper, diced
- 2 cloves of garlic, minced
- 2 cups fresh spinach or arugula

Directions:

- In a mixing bowl, whisk together the eggs, milk, salt, and pepper.
- Heat the olive oil in a large skillet over medium-high heat.
- Add the onion, red bell pepper, and garlic and sauté until softened.
- Add the spinach or arugula and cook until wilted.
- Pour the egg mixture into the skillet and stir gently to combine with the vegetables.
- Reduce the heat to medium-low and cook until the bottom is set.
- Sprinkle the grated Parmesan cheese over the top of the frittata.
- Place the skillet under the broiler for a couple of minutes, or until the top is golden brown and set.

- Slice and serve the frittata warm, garnished with additional herbs or a sprinkle of Parmesan cheese if desired.

This recipe is a great way to include a variety of vegetables, which are an important part of a healthy diet for those with Ulcerative colitis. The egg is a good source of protein, and it's also easy to digest. Spinach and arugula are low in FODMAPs, which is a group of fermentable carbohydrates that may cause symptoms for people with Ulcerative colitis. The Parmesan cheese can be omitted or replaced with other cheese that you can eat.

As always, it is important to check with your doctor or a registered dietitian to see what specific foods and dietary restrictions are best for you. They may also provide a list of foods that you should avoid or limit and give you advice on how to manage your condition through diet and nutrition.

PART THREE

MEAL PLAN

I would like to reiterate that everyone's dietary needs are unique and this meal plan may not be appropriate for everyone. Additionally, it's always best to consult with a dietitian or nutritionist to develop a personalized meal plan that takes into account your specific needs and dietary restrictions. Also, it's important to note that some people with Ulcerative Colitis may have food triggers that they need to avoid, so it's important to be aware of your own body and listen to it.

It's also important to mention that a diet high in fiber can be beneficial for people with Ulcerative Colitis, as it can help reduce inflammation and regulate bowel movements. However, it's also important to introduce fiber gradually and drink plenty of water to avoid gas and bloating. Additionally, a diet that includes lean protein, healthy fats, and plenty of fruits and vegetables can also be beneficial.

It's important to note that the meal plan below is just an example and should be adjusted to fit individual needs and dietary restrictions.
Additionally, it's recommended to check with a healthcare professional or a registered dietitian to make sure that the plan is suitable for you.

Here is an example of a healthy meal plan for a person with ulcerative colitis:

MEAL PLAN FOR ULCERATIVE COLITIS PATIENTS			
	BREAKFAST	**LUNCH**	**DINNER**
MONDAY	Oatmeal with blueberries and almond milk	Grilled chicken breast with quinoa and steamed vegetables	Baked salmon with sweet potato and green beans
TUESDAY	Greek yogurt with honey and granola	Turkey and cheese sandwich on whole wheat bread with a side of carrot sticks	Spinach and ricotta stuffed chicken breast with brown rice and steamed broccoli
WEDNESDAY	Scrambled eggs with spinach and mushrooms	Tuna salad sandwich on whole wheat bread with a side of fruit	Baked turkey meatballs with whole wheat pasta and marinara sauce
THURSDAY	Smoothie bowl made with Greek yogurt, berries, and spinach	Grilled chicken Caesar salad	Chicken and vegetable stir-fry with brown rice
FRIDAY	Avocado toast on whole wheat bread	Turkey chili with a side of green salad	Grilled shrimp with roasted vegetables and quinoa
SATURDAY	French toast made with whole wheat bread and topped with fruit	Turkey and cheese wrap with a side of sweet potato fries	Baked cod with a side of roasted vegetables
SUNDAY	Scrambled eggs with diced tomatoes and onions	Grilled chicken breast with a side of brown rice and steamed vegetables	Vegetable lasagna with a side of green salad

CONCLUSION

In conclusion, Ulcerative Colitis is a chronic inflammatory bowel disease that affects the large intestine. The journey of living with UC can be difficult and challenging, but it is important to remember that you are not alone. The exact cause of UC is still not known, but it is believed to be a combination of genetic and environmental factors. The symptoms of UC can vary from person to person and can range from mild to severe. They include diarrhea, abdominal pain, rectal bleeding, weight loss, fatigue, and anemia. These symptoms can greatly impact a person's quality of life, making it hard to carry out day-to-day activities.

Treatment for UC involves a combination of medication, lifestyle changes, and in some cases, surgery. Medications such as aminosalicylates, corticosteroids, and immunomodulators can help reduce inflammation and ease symptoms. Lifestyle changes such as a healthy diet and regular exercise can also help manage symptoms. Surgery, such as the removal of the colon, may be necessary in severe cases.

While there is currently no cure for UC, many people are able to manage their symptoms and lead fulfilling lives with proper treatment. It is important for those with UC to work closely with their healthcare provider to develop an individualized treatment plan that works for them. It's also important to seek emotional support as living with a chronic illness can be emotionally taxing as well. Joining a support group or seeing a therapist can be very beneficial.

In summary, Ulcerative Colitis is a chronic condition that can be challenging to live with, but with the right treatment, support and positive attitude, it is possible to lead a fulfilling life. It's important to remember that you are not alone in this journey and there are many resources available to help you manage your symptoms and improve your quality of life.